DISABILITY CARE GUIDE

FOR PARENTS AND CAREGIVERS

Dr. A. MITRA, MBBS, MD, DMI.

Disclaimer:

The information provided in this book, "Disability Care Guide: For Parents and Caregivers," is intended for educational purposes only. While every effort has been made to ensure accuracy and relevance, readers are advised to consult healthcare professionals for personalized advice and treatment options tailored to individual circumstances. The author and publisher disclaim any liability arising directly or indirectly from the use or application of the contents of this book.

DEDICATION

This is a tribute to the heroes in all caregivers including parents and families who, with their ceaseless love, resilience, and commitment, provide individuals with disability the strength to overcome obstacles and flourish. The steadfast bravery and perseverance of these heroes serve as an inspiration to us all.

CONTENTS

- Understanding Different Types of Seizures and Their Triggers
- Recognizing Signs and Symptoms of an Impending Seizure
- Creating a Safe Environment for Individuals with Seizures
- First Aid Procedures for Seizures
- Post-Seizure Care and Support

- Different Types of Home Healthcare Professionals (Nurses, Physical Therapists, Occupational Therapists, etc.)
- Roles and Responsibilities of Home Healthcare Professionals
- Effective Communication with Home Healthcare Professionals
- Coordinating Care Plans and Sharing Information
- Advocating for the Needs of the Individual with a Disability

- Types of Physical Disabilities and Their Impact on Daily Life (Spinal Cord Injuries, Amputations, etc.)
- Specific Care Needs for Different Physical Disabilities
- Pain Management Strategies for Individuals with Chronic Pain

- Transition Planning and Considerations for Aging with a Disability
- Technological Advancements and Assistive Technologies for Future Care
- Financial Planning and Funding Options for Long-Term Care

ACKNOWLEDGMENTS

I extend heartfelt gratitude to all who contributed to "Disability Care Guide: For Parents and Caregivers." Thanks to the courageous individual caregivers and families for sharing their experiences. Deep appreciation to healthcare professionals, therapists, educators, and researchers for their dedication. Special thanks to colleagues, friends, and mentors for their unwavering support and feedback. Gratitude also to the publishing team for their hard work. This book is a testament to a compassionate community dedicated to empowering individuals with disability and fostering inclusivity.

Thank you all.

Dr. A. Mitra

1. UNDERSTANDING DISABILITY

This chapter is our roadmap to the world of disabilities. We will explore different types of disabilities, what might cause them, and how they can impact people's lives. Remember, everyone is unique, and disabilities are like different abilities people use to navigate the world. Let us dive in.

Major Categories of Disabilities

Imagine a toolbox filled with various tools. A hammer helps you build, a screwdriver fixes things, and a wrench tightens connections. Similarly, disabilities are like different abilities people use to experience the world. Here are some major categories:

- **Physical Disabilities:** These affect someone's body, making it harder to move or perform daily activities. People with physical disabilities might use wheelchairs, crutches, canes, or prosthetics (artificial limbs) to help them get around and be independent. Some examples include:
    - **Spinal Cord Injuries:** Damage to the spinal cord can affect movement and sensation in the body.
    - **Muscular Dystrophy:** A group of diseases that weaken muscles over time.
    - **Arthritis:** Painful inflammation of joints that can limit mobility.

- **Sensory Disabilities:** These affect how someone perceives the world through their senses. People with sensory disabilities might use assistive technologies or strategies to navigate their environment. Here are some examples:
  - **Visual Impairments:** This can range from blurry vision to complete blindness. People might use white canes, guide dogs, or screen readers (software that reads text aloud) to navigate.
  - **Hearing Impairments:** This can range from mild hearing loss to complete deafness. People might use hearing aids, sign language, or lipreading to communicate.
  - **Deaf-blindness:** This is a combination of vision and hearing loss. People who are deafblind use specialized communication methods and rely heavily on touch and other senses.

- **Intellectual Disabilities:** These affect a person's cognitive development and ability to learn new skills. They might need extra support with daily tasks, learning concepts, or social interaction. Some examples include:
  - **Down Syndrome:** A genetic condition that affects development in various areas.

- o **Fragile X Syndrome:** A genetic condition that can cause intellectual disabilities and social challenges.
- o **Autism Spectrum Disorder (ASD):** A developmental condition characterized by social interaction difficulties and repetitive behaviors.

- **Developmental Disabilities:** These are disabilities that appear early in childhood and can affect a person's physical or intellectual development. These might overlap with other categories. An example is cerebral palsy, which affects movement and muscle control.

- **Mental Health Conditions:** These are conditions that affect a person's emotional and mental well-being. Examples include anxiety, depression, and bipolar disorder.

Causes and Risk Factors

There are many reasons why someone might have a disability. Some disabilities are present from birth due to genetic conditions, like Down syndrome or chromosomal abnormalities. Others may develop later in life due to accidents, illnesses like meningitis, or exposure to toxins during pregnancy. Some disabilities can also be a combination of factors.

The Impact of Disabilities

Having a disability can present challenges in certain aspects of life. For example:

- **Physical Impact:** A person with a physical disability might need help with daily tasks like bathing, dressing, or preparing meals.
- **Social Impact:** Someone with a sensory disability might find it harder to socialize or participate in group activities.
- **Emotional Impact:** A person with a mental health condition might experience depression, anxiety, or difficulty managing emotions.

Remember: It is important to focus on the abilities. While disabilities can create challenges, they do not define who someone is. With support and understanding, people with disabilities can live fulfilling and joyful lives. They can excel in school, pursue careers, maintain strong relationships, and actively contribute to their communities.

The Takeaway:

This chapter has just opened the door to the world of disabilities. By understanding different categories, causes, and impacts, we can build a more inclusive world where everyone feels valued and empowered.

2. DISABILITY RIGHTS AND LEGISLATION

This chapter delves into the fight for equality for people with disabilities. We will explore the history of disability rights movements, key legislation that protects these rights, and the important role caregivers play in upholding them.

History of Disability Rights Movements

For many years, people with disabilities faced discrimination and exclusion. Thankfully, courageous individuals and organizations launched disability rights movements to fight for equality. These movements played a crucial role in raising awareness and influencing legislation.

Key Disability Rights Legislation

Many countries have enacted laws to protect the rights of people with disabilities. Here are some prominent examples:

- **The Americans with Disabilities Act (ADA):** A landmark law in the United States that prohibits discrimination against people with disabilities in employment, education, public services, and transportation. It requires public spaces to be accessible, meaning people with disabilities can easily enter and use them.

- **The Individuals with Disabilities Education Act (IDEA):** This U.S. law guarantees free and appropriate public education for all children with disabilities. It ensures they receive the support and services they need to succeed in school.

Rights of People with Disabilities

Disability rights legislation protects various rights for people with disabilities, including:

- **Employment:** People with disabilities have the right to be considered for jobs based on their qualifications, not their disability. Employers must provide reasonable accommodations, such as modified workstations or assistive technology, to help them perform their duties.
- **Education:** Children with disabilities have the right to a quality education in the least restrictive environment possible. This means they should be educated alongside their peers without disabilities whenever possible, with appropriate support services provided.
- **Access:** Public spaces and buildings must be accessible, including features like ramps, elevators, and accessible restrooms. Transportation systems should also be accessible to ensure people with disabilities can get around independently.
- **Participation:** People with disabilities have the right to participate fully in their communities. This

includes involvement in social activities, government programs, and civic engagement.

The Role of Caregivers in Upholding Disability Rights

As a caregiver, you play a vital role in upholding the rights of the individual you support. Here is how you can make a difference:

- **Be Informed:** Educate yourself about disability rights legislation and resources available in your area. Knowledge is power.
- **Empowerment:** Encourage the person you support to make their own choices and participate in decision-making whenever possible.
  - o This fosters independence and a sense of control.
- **Advocate on Their Behalf:** If necessary, advocate for their rights and ensure they receive the support and services they are entitled to under disability rights legislation.
  - o Be their voice when needed.
- **Promote Inclusion:** Work towards creating an inclusive environment where the individual feels valued, respected, and empowered to participate fully in society.
  - o Celebrate their abilities and contributions.

Remember: Disability rights legislation is a powerful

tool for creating a more just and equitable world for everyone. By understanding these rights and taking action, we can ensure that people with disabilities have the opportunity to reach their full potential.

3. COMMUNICATION AND INTERACTION

Communication is like a bridge, connecting us and allowing us to understand each other. When someone has a disability, this bridge might need some adjustments, but the goal remains the same: to connect, share ideas, and build strong relationships.

Why Does Effective Communication Matter?

Clear communication is essential for everyone, but it is especially important when interacting with people with disabilities. It helps to:

- **Reduce Frustration:** Miscommunication can be frustrating for everyone. Effective communication minimizes confusion and ensures everyone is on the same page.
- **Build Trust and Rapport:** When we can understand each other, trust and rapport grow. This fosters positive relationships.
- **Empowerment:** Effective communication empowers people with disabilities to express themselves, make choices, and participate fully in life.

Communication Strategies for Different Needs

People communicate in diverse ways, and disabilities

can sometimes affect communication styles. Here are some tips for interacting effectively with different disabilities:

- **Visual Impairments:** People with visual impairments might rely on verbal descriptions, sound cues, or touch to understand their environment.
    - o Describe your surroundings clearly, and ask before offering physical guidance.
- **Hearing Impairments:** Some people with hearing impairments rely on sign language, lipreading, or assistive listening devices.
    - o Face-to-face communication and minimizing background noise are crucial. Be patient and willing to repeat information if needed.
- **Speech Impairments:** People with speech impairments might use alternative communication methods like assistive technology (voice synthesizers, picture boards) or writing.
    - o Be patient and allow them ample time to express themselves using their preferred method.
- **Intellectual Disabilities:** People with intellectual disabilities might benefit from clear, concise language and breaking down information into smaller steps.
    - o Visual aids and focusing on one topic at a time can enhance comprehension.

- **Autism Spectrum Disorder (ASD):** Individuals with ASD might have challenges with social interaction and communication.
  - o Respect their preferred level of interaction and avoid overwhelming them with too much information at once. Focus on clear, literal communication and be mindful of nonverbal cues.

Understanding Non-Verbal Communication

Communication is not just about words. Non-verbal cues like facial expressions, body language, and gestures also play a significant role. Pay attention to these nonverbal signals to gain a deeper understanding of the person you are communicating with.

Active Listening

Active listening is the foundation of good communication. It involves paying close attention to both verbal and nonverbal cues. Here are some tips for active listening:

- **Give Your Full Attention:** Minimize distractions and focus entirely on the person you are communicating with.
- **Show Empathy:** Try to understand their perspective and acknowledge their feelings.

- **Ask Clarifying Questions:** If something is unclear, ask polite questions to ensure you understand their message accurately.
- **Avoid Interrupting:** Allow them to finish their thoughts before responding.

Respectful Language Matters

The words we use have power. Here are some guidelines for respectful language:

- **Person-First Language:** Refer to individuals by their name first, emphasizing their personhood rather than their disability (e.g., say "person with a disability" instead of "disabled person").
- **Positive and Inclusive Language:** Avoid using patronizing or stereotypical language. Treat everyone with dignity and respect.

Assistive Communication Tools

Technology can be a powerful bridge for communication. Here are some assistive communication ideas that can be helpful:

- **AAC Devices:** Augmentative and Alternative Communication (AAC) devices can help people with speech impairments communicate using pictures, symbols, or synthesized speech.

- **Sign Language:** Learning basic sign language can be a valuable tool for communication with people who are deaf or hard of hearing.

Remember: Communication is a two-way street. By being patient, adaptable, and open to learning new communication styles, you can build strong and meaningful relationships with people who have disabilities. Let us work together to create a world where everyone feels heard, valued, and understood.

4. PERSONAL CARE ROUTINES

Taking care of ourselves, from brushing our teeth to washing our hair, is essential for good health and feeling our best. This chapter focuses on personal care routines, with special considerations for people with disabilities. Remember, everyone deserves to feel clean and comfortable.

Why Does Personal Hygiene Matter?

Just like everyone else, people with disabilities need good personal hygiene to stay healthy and prevent infections. Regular bathing, washing hands, and taking care of skin helps to:

- **Reduce the risk of infections:** Good hygiene removes germs that can cause illness.
- **Maintain skin health:** Clean skin is less prone to irritation and rashes.
- **Boost confidence and well-being:** Feeling clean and fresh can improve self-esteem and overall well-being.

Making Bath Time Easier

Bathing and showering can be challenging for some people with disabilities. Here are some tips to make it a safe and comfortable experience:

- **Grab Bars and Shower Seats:** Installing grab bars in the bathroom and using a shower seat can provide extra support and stability.
- **Hand-Held Shower Heads:** These offer more control and flexibility compared to fixed showerheads.
- **Bath Lifts:** For people with limited mobility, bath lifts can safely transfer them in and out of the bathtub.
- **Always maintain a comfortable water temperature to avoid scalding.**

Taking Care of our Skin

People with certain disabilities might be more prone to skin problems. Here are some tips for healthy skin:

- **Use gentle cleansers and moisturizers:** Harsh soaps can dry out the skin. Opt for fragrance-free and gentle products.
- **Regular skin checks:** Look for any signs of irritation, redness, or pressure sores. Early detection helps prevent complications.
- **Proper drying:** Pay attention to areas with skin folds, like between toes or under arms, to prevent moisture buildup and potential infections.

Dressing Techniques for Limited Mobility

Getting dressed can be difficult for some people with disabilities. Here are some tips to make it easier:

- **Loose-fitting clothing:** Choose clothes that are easy to put on and take off, like clothes with zippers or slip-on styles.
- **Dress in stages:** Sit down while putting on clothes, especially pants and socks.
- **Assistive devices:** Dresser extenders, long-handled shoe horns, and button hooks can make dressing more manageable.

Toileting Assistance and Catheter Care (if applicable)

For some people with disabilities, toileting might require assistance. If you are a caregiver, it is important to be trained on proper techniques to ensure privacy, dignity, and hygiene.

Catheter care requires specific instructions and hygiene practices to prevent infections. Always follow healthcare professional guidance for catheter use and maintenance.

Considerations for Specific Disabilities

When it comes to personal care routines, it is crucial to

consider the specific needs of each person. Here are some general considerations for different disabilities:

- **Physical Disabilities:** People with limited mobility might require assistance with bathing, dressing, and toileting.
- **Visual Impairments:** Provide clear verbal instructions and descriptions during personal care routines.
- **Intellectual Disabilities:** Break down tasks into smaller steps and offer positive reinforcement.

Remember: Personal care is a collaborative effort. Communication, respect for privacy, and ensuring comfort are key to establishing successful personal care routines. By working together, we can empower people with disabilities to maintain good hygiene and live independently to the greatest extent possible.

5. SAFE TRANSFERS AND MOBILITY

Moving around safely and independently is crucial for everyone. This chapter focuses on safe mobility and transfer techniques for people with disabilities, along with helpful equipment and modifications to create a more accessible environment. Remember, independence and confidence go hand in hand.

Why Does Safe Mobility Matter?

Being able to move around safely is essential for independence and well-being. It allows people to:

- **Perform daily activities:** Moving around safely is necessary for basic tasks like getting dressed, using the bathroom, or preparing meals.
- **Maintain physical health:** Regular movement helps prevent muscle stiffness, improves circulation, and promotes overall health.
- **Boost self-esteem and confidence:** The ability to move independently fosters a sense of control and well-being.

Making Transfers Safe and Smooth

Transferring from one position to another, like from a bed to a wheelchair, requires proper techniques to ensure safety and prevent injury. Here is a general overview:

- **Standing Transfers:** These involve moving from a sitting position to standing. Use strong support and ensure proper leg positioning for balance.
- **Sitting Transfers:** These involve moving from standing to sitting. Provide a stable surface to sit on and support as needed.
- **Always assess the individual's strength and ability before attempting a transfer.**

Your Mobility Partner: Assistive Devices

Assistive mobility devices can significantly improve a person's independence and ability to move around safely. Here are some common examples:

- **Wheelchairs:** These provide mobility for people with limited leg function. Different types cater to various needs.
- **Canes:** Offer single-point support for balance and stability while walking.
- **Walkers:** Provide more support than canes, with four legs for increased stability.
- **Gait belts:** These belts can be used by caregivers to provide additional support during transfers or walking.

Gait Training and Safe Walking

Gait training can help individuals with disabilities improve their walking ability and balance. A physical or occupational therapist can develop a personalized program based on specific needs. Here are some general tips for safe walking:

- **Wear appropriate footwear:** Shoes should be well-fitting with good traction to prevent slipping.
- **Maintain good posture:** Stand tall with shoulders back and head held high for better balance.
- **Take your time and focus on each step:** Do not rush, and pay attention to your surroundings.

Home Modifications for Improved Mobility

Simple modifications can make a big difference in a person's ability to move around safely at home. Here are some ideas:

- **Ramps:** Install ramps for entryways or steps to eliminate barriers.
- **Grab bars:** Adding grab bars in bathrooms, near stairs, and along hallways provides extra support for balance.
- **Widened doorways:** Wider doorways allow for easier passage with wheelchairs or other mobility devices.
- **Lowered light switches and cabinet knobs:** Making these controls easier to reach promotes independence.

Safety Considerations During Transfers and Mobility

Safety is paramount during transfers and mobility activities. Here are some important considerations:

- **Clear the area:** Remove any obstacles that could cause tripping or falls.
- **Proper body mechanics:** Use proper lifting techniques to protect yourself and the person you are assisting from injury.
- **Communicate clearly:** Talk through each step of the transfer process to ensure understanding and prevent confusion.
- **Always prioritize safety:** If you are unsure about a transfer, do not hesitate to ask for help from a healthcare professional.

Remember: Mobility and safe transfers are essential for independence. By using proper techniques, assistive devices, and making modifications to the environment, we can empower people with disabilities to move around safely and confidently in their daily lives.

6. NUTRITION AND MEAL PREPARATION

Food is like fuel for our bodies. Just like everyone's unique, nutritional needs can vary depending on age, health conditions, and abilities. This chapter explores healthy eating for people with disabilities, focusing on adapting meals and kitchens to promote independence and well-being.

Why Does Good Nutrition Matter?

Eating a balanced diet with plenty of fruits, vegetables, whole grains, and lean protein is crucial for everyone's health. For people with disabilities, proper nutrition is even more important because it can:

- **Boost energy levels:** Nutritious food provides the energy needed for daily activities and overall well-being.
- **Maintain a healthy weight:** A balanced diet helps manage weight, which can be especially important for some disabilities.
- **Support healing and recovery:** Proper nutrition helps the body heal from illness or surgery, which can be more common for some people with disabilities.

Different Dietary Needs

People with disabilities might have specific dietary

needs based on their condition. Here are some common examples:

- **Diabetic Diets:** These diets focus on managing blood sugar levels through controlled carbohydrate intake.
- **Dysphagia Diets:** These diets involve modified textures (like puréed food or thickened liquids) for people with swallowing difficulties.
- **Lactose Intolerance:** This requires limiting or avoiding dairy products due to difficulty digesting lactose, a sugar found in milk.

Shopping and Meal Planning

Planning meals and creating a grocery list ahead of time is essential for healthy eating, especially with specific dietary needs. Here are some tips:

- **Consult a healthcare professional or registered dietitian:** They can help create a personalized meal plan that addresses specific nutritional requirements.
- **Plan meals around easy-to-prepare options:** Choose recipes that are simple to follow and do not require extensive cooking techniques.
- **Read food labels carefully:** Be mindful of ingredients and nutritional information, especially for people with specific dietary restrictions.

Adaptive Techniques and Modifications for Kitchen

A well-organized and accessible kitchen can make meal preparation safer and easier for people with disabilities. Here are some considerations:

- **Lower shelves and cabinets:** Make frequently used items easily reachable.
- **Countertop extensions:** These can provide extra work surface area for people who use wheelchairs.
- **Adaptive utensils:** Utensils with built-up handles or weighted grips can be easier to hold.
- **Assistive technology:** Voice-activated appliances or specially designed cutting boards can simplify tasks.

Safe Food Handling and Meal Preparation

Safe food handling is essential to prevent foodborne illnesses. Here are some key practices:

- **Wash hands thoroughly:** Always wash your hands properly with soap and water before and after handling food.
- **Cook food to proper temperatures:** Use a food thermometer to ensure meats and poultry reach safe internal temperatures.

- **Store leftovers properly:** Refrigerate or freeze leftovers within two hours of cooking to prevent bacterial growth.

Feeding Techniques for Different Needs

Some people with disabilities might require assistance with eating. Here are some feeding techniques to consider:

- **Spoon-feeding:** This involves slowly placing small bites of food on the tongue and ensuring safe swallowing.
- **Thickened Liquids:** These can be easier to swallow for people with dysphagia. Thickening agents are available commercially or through a healthcare professional.
- **Adaptive feeding tools:** Specialized spoons, cups, or plates can make eating easier for people with limited hand function.

Remember: Healthy eating is a cornerstone of well-being for everyone. By understanding dietary needs, planning meals effectively, and adapting kitchens and techniques, we can empower people with disabilities to enjoy nutritious and delicious meals independently whenever possible.

7. ENCOURAGING SELF-CARE SKILLS

Imagine a bird learning to fly. It takes practice, encouragement, and confidence to spread its wings and soar. This chapter focuses on fostering independence in people with disabilities by promoting self-care skills. By taking small steps and celebrating successes, we can all reach new heights.

Why is Independence Important?

Independence means being able to take care of yourself and make your own choices. It fosters a sense of control, dignity, and self-esteem. Here is why promoting independence is crucial:

- **Increased Confidence:** The ability to do things for themselves boosts confidence and self-worth in people with disabilities.
- **Improved Quality of Life:** Independence allows people to participate more actively in daily life and pursue their interests.
- **Empowerment:** Learning self-care skills empowers people with disabilities to make choices and manage their lives.

Identifying Individual Goals and Capabilities

The path to independence is unique for everyone. The first step is identifying individual goals and capabilities.

Here is how:

- **Work Together:** Collaborate with the person with a disability and their healthcare team to determine realistic goals.
- **Consider Strengths:** Focus on existing strengths and abilities as a foundation for building new skills.
- **Start Small:** Set achievable goals that can be broken down into manageable steps.

Breaking Down the Tasks into Achievable Steps

Big tasks can seem overwhelming. Breaking them down into smaller, more manageable steps makes them less daunting and easier to accomplish. Here is how:

- **Create a Checklist:** List the steps involved in a task, breaking it down into smaller, achievable actions.
- **Practice Makes Progress:** Encourage regular practice of self-care skills to build confidence and mastery.
- **Celebrate Milestones:** Acknowledge and celebrate even small victories to maintain motivation.

Using Adaptive Equipment and Techniques

Adaptive equipment and techniques can make a big difference in promoting independence. Here are some examples:

- **Dressing aids:** Long-handled shoehorn, button hooks, or zipper pulls can make dressing easier.
- **Shower chairs and grab bars:** These provide support and stability in the bathroom.
- **Meal preparation tools:** Rocker knives, adaptive cutting boards, or electric can openers can simplify meal prep.

Building Confidence and Self-Esteem

Confidence is like a muscle that gets stronger with exercise. Here are some ways to build confidence in individuals with disabilities:

- **Positive Reinforcement:** Offer encouragement, praise effort, and celebrate achievements, no matter how small.
- **Focus on Abilities:** Highlight strengths and capabilities rather than limitations.
- **Promote Choice and Control:** Allow individuals to make choices whenever possible, fostering a sense of control and autonomy.

Remember: The journey towards independence is a collaborative effort. By working together, setting achievable goals, and providing encouragement and support, we can empower people with disabilities to develop self-care skills, build confidence, and soar towards a life of greater independence.

8. MEDICATION MANAGEMENT

Medications play a crucial role in managing many health conditions. This chapter equips you with the knowledge to manage medications safely and effectively, whether for yourself or someone you care for. Remember, medication safety is key to good health.

Why Does Safe Medication Use Matter?

Taking medications correctly is essential for getting the most benefit and avoiding potential harm. Here is why safe medication use matters:

- **Improved Health Outcomes:** Proper medication use helps control symptoms and manage health conditions effectively.
- **Reduced Risk of Side Effects:** Understanding medications and taking them correctly minimizes the risk of unwanted side effects.
- **Peace of Mind:** Knowing you are managing medications safely promotes a sense of control and well-being.

Understanding Different Medication Types

Medications come in various forms, each with its own administration method. Here is a quick breakdown:

- **Tablets:** These are solid pills swallowed whole or crushed (depending on the medication).
- **Capsules:** Similar to tablets, but often contain powder or liquid medication.
- **Liquids:** Syrups or suspensions, often used for children or people with swallowing difficulties.
- **Injections:** Medications injected into the muscle, fatty tissue, or bloodstream using a needle and syringe.
- **Inhalers:** Deliver medication directly to the lungs through mouth inhalation.

Handling and Storing Medications

Safe medication handling and storage are crucial to prevent misuse or accidents. Here are some key practices:

- **Read Labels Carefully:** Always double-check the medication name, dosage, and expiry date before taking it.
- **Store Medications Properly:** Keep them in their original containers, in a cool, dry place, out of reach of children and pets.
- **Dispose of Expired Medications Safely:** Do not throw medications in the trash. Ask your pharmacist about proper disposal methods.

Recognizing Side Effects and Interactions

Medications can sometimes cause side effects, which are unwanted reactions to the medication. Here is what to watch for:

- **Common Side Effects:** These are usually mild and temporary, like drowsiness or upset stomach.
- **Serious Side Effects:** These are less common but can be dangerous. Report these to your doctor immediately.
- **Medication Interactions:** Some medications can interact with each other, causing unwanted effects. Inform your doctor about all medications you are taking, including over-the-counter drugs and supplements.

Medication Recordkeeping

Keeping a medication record helps ensure taking medications correctly and on schedule. Here is what to include in the record:

- **Medication Name and Dosage:** Write down the name, strength, and dosage of each medication.
- **Frequency:** Record how often you need to take each medication (e.g., daily, twice a day).
- **Notes:** Include any special instructions or potential side effects.

Partnering with Healthcare Providers

Your doctor or pharmacist is your partner in safe medication management. Here is how to work effectively with them:

- **Ask Questions:** Do not hesitate to ask questions about your medications, side effects, or interactions.
- **Report Changes:** Inform your doctor about any changes in your health or new medications you start taking.
- **Schedule Regular Checkups:** Attend regular doctor appointments to review your medications and overall health.

Remember: Taking charge of your medication management empowers you to be an active participant in your healthcare. By understanding medications, handling them safely, and working with your healthcare providers, you can ensure you get the most benefit from your medications and stay healthy.

9. BOWEL AND BLADDER MANAGEMENT

Our bodies do amazing things. This chapter dives into normal bowel and bladder function, and how to manage situations where things might not work perfectly. It also covers ostomy care, which helps people whose digestive system has undergone changes. Remember, everyone deserves to feel confident and in control.

Normal Bowel and Bladder Function

- **Bowels:** We typically have bowel movements (BM) once a day, though this can vary. Stool (poop) should be soft and easy to pass.
- **Bladder:** The bladder stores urine (pee) until we are ready to use the restroom. We usually urinate several times a day.

Understanding and Managing Incontinence

Sometimes, accidents happen. Incontinence means having difficulty controlling your bladder or bowels. Here is a breakdown:

- **Types of Incontinence:** There are different types, like urinary incontinence (leakage of pee) or fecal incontinence (leakage of stool).
- **Management Strategies:** Depending on the type and cause, incontinence can be managed with

lifestyle changes, exercises, medications, or absorbent products (adult diapers).

Catheter Care

Catheters are thin tubes inserted into the bladder to drain urine. They might be temporary or long-term, depending on the situation. Here is a quick overview:

- **Types of Catheters:** There are different types, like Foley catheters (inserted through the urethra) or suprapubic catheters (inserted through the belly).
- **Catheter Care:** Proper cleaning and maintenance are crucial to prevent infections. Always follow healthcare professional instructions.

Stoma Care

An ostomy is a surgical procedure that creates an opening (stoma) on the abdomen to divert waste products. People with ostomy might use pouches to collect waste. Here is a basic understanding:

- **Types of Ostomy Systems:** There are different ostomy systems depending on the type of surgery.
- **Cleaning and Maintenance:** Regular cleaning and emptying of pouches is essential for hygiene and preventing skin problems. Follow healthcare professional instructions for specific care.

Promoting Healthy Habits

Here are some tips to keep your bowel and bladder healthy:

- **Stay Hydrated:** Drink plenty of fluids throughout the day to promote healthy urine flow and prevent constipation.
- **Fiber Up:** Eat plenty of fiber-rich foods like fruits, vegetables, and whole grains to aid digestion.
- **Healthy Bathroom Habits:** Go to the bathroom when you feel the urge and avoid holding it in for long periods.
- **Pelvic Floor Exercises:** These exercises can strengthen muscles that support bladder control.

Remember: You are not alone. Bowel and bladder issues are common, and there are many ways to manage them. By understanding normal function, incontinence, catheters, ostomy care, and healthy habits, you can take charge of your well-being and live life confidently. Always consult your healthcare professional for personalized guidance and support.

10. PROTECTING SKIN

Our skin is our body's largest organ, protecting us from the outside world. This chapter focuses on the importance of skin care for people with limited mobility, who are more prone to pressure injuries (bed sores). By following simple strategies, we can keep skin healthy and prevent complications. Remember, healthy skin is happy skin.

Why Does Skin Care Matter for Limited Mobility?

People who sit or lie down for extended periods are more at risk of developing pressure injuries. Here is why skin care is crucial:

- **Pressure Hurts:** Constant pressure on specific areas can reduce blood flow, leading to skin breakdown and pressure injuries.
- **Infection Risks:** Open wounds from pressure injuries are susceptible to infection, which can be serious.
- **Pain and Discomfort:** Pressure injuries can be painful and uncomfortable, affecting quality of life.

Recognizing Signs of Skin Breakdown

Early detection is key to preventing pressure injuries. Here is what to watch for:

- **Redness:** Persistent redness on skin that does not fade when pressure is removed.
- **Warmth:** Skin that feels warm to the touch in a specific area.
- **Pain or Tenderness:** Skin that feels painful or tender when touched.
- **Changes in Skin Color:** Skin that becomes darker or purple may indicate a serious pressure injury.

Techniques for Skin Care and Prevention

Simple skin care practices can make a big difference. Here are some helpful tips:

- **Regular Skin Checks:** Inspect the skin daily for any signs of redness, warmth, or breakdown.
- **Moisturizing:** Use a fragrance-free moisturizer to keep skin hydrated and supple.
- **Frequent Position Changes:** Shift positions every two hours for people who sit or lie down for extended periods.
- **Pressure Relief Devices:** Use specialized cushions, pillows, or mattresses designed to redistribute pressure.

Proper Use of Positioning Aids

Positioning aids can help prevent pressure injuries by distributing weight more evenly. Here are some examples:

- **Pressure-reducing cushions:** These cushions are designed to reduce pressure points when sitting in a wheelchair or chair.
- **Turning pillows:** These pillows help with turning and repositioning in bed.
- **Heel protectors:** These protect heels from pressure and skin breakdown.

Nutritional Considerations

Good nutrition plays a vital role in skin health. Here is what to keep in mind:

- **Stay Hydrated:** Drinking plenty of fluids helps keep skin hydrated and promotes overall health.
- **Protein Power:** Protein is essential for building and repairing skin tissues. Include lean protein sources in your diet.
- **Essential Vitamins:** Vitamins A, C, and E are crucial for skin health. Ensure a balanced diet rich in fruits, vegetables, and whole grains.

Remember: Skin care is a collaborative effort. By working together, following these strategies, and seeking professional guidance if needed, we can keep skin healthy and prevent pressure injuries, promoting comfort and well-being for people with limited mobility.

11. HOUSEHOLD TASK MANAGEMENT

A clean and organized home is a happy home. This chapter explores practical strategies for managing household tasks like laundry, light housekeeping, and errands, with a focus on making them accessible for people with disabilities. Remember, a little adaptation can go a long way.

Why Does a Clean Home Matter?

Keeping your living space clean and organized has many benefits:

- **Improved Health:** A clean environment helps reduce the spread of germs and allergens, promoting good health.
- **Reduced Stress:** Living in a cluttered space can feel overwhelming. A clean and organized home fosters a sense of calm and well-being.
- **Increased Independence:** The ability to manage household tasks can empower people with disabilities and contribute to a greater sense of independence.

Laundry Techniques and Considerations

Laundry might seem like a chore, but there are ways to make it easier. Here are some tips for people with disabilities:

- **Front-loading washing machines:** These can be easier to load and unload than top-loading machines, especially for people with limited bending ability.
- **Assistive devices:** Grabber tools or laundry baskets with wheels can make laundry tasks less strenuous.
- **Planning and prioritizing:** Wash similar clothes together, and plan laundry days based on ability and energy levels.

Light Housekeeping with Accessibility in Mind

Keeping your home clean does not require backbreaking effort. Here are some accessibility considerations for light housekeeping tasks:

- **Cleaning tools with long handles:** These can help reach higher areas without excessive bending or straining.
- **Lightweight vacuum cleaners:** These are easier to maneuver for people with limited mobility.
- **Elevated cleaning supplies:** Store cleaning supplies on lower shelves or use organizers to avoid reaching for high places.

Planning and Completing Errands

Errands are a necessary part of life. Here are some tips for managing them with limited mobility:

- **Planning and prioritizing:** Make a list of errands and prioritize them. Can some errands be combined?
- **Online shopping and delivery services:** Take advantage of online options to minimize trips to the store.
- **Curbside pickup:** Many stores offer curbside pickup for online orders. Call ahead to confirm availability.

Time Management

There never seem to be enough hours in the day. Here are some time management tips for household tasks:

- **Create a schedule:** Break down tasks into smaller, manageable chunks and schedule them throughout the week.
- **Delegate tasks:** If possible, share household responsibilities.
- **Focus on what matters most:** Prioritize essential tasks and do not be afraid to let go of less important things.

Utilizing Resources for Household Assistance

Do not be afraid to ask for help. There are many resources available to assist with household tasks:

- **Professional cleaning services:** Consider hiring professional cleaners if needed.
- **In-home care services:** These services can provide assistance with various household tasks.
- **Friends and family:** Lean on your support network for help with errands or occasional chores.

Remember: Maintaining a clean and organized home is an ongoing process. By adapting tasks to your abilities, utilizing time management strategies, and seeking help when needed, you can create a comfortable and livable environment that promotes independence and well-being for everyone.

12. ACCESSIBLE TRANSPORTATION

Imagine a world where everyone can go where they want, when they want. This chapter focuses on transportation and community access for people with disabilities, exploring options like public transit, adapted vehicles, and travel assistance services. Remember, exploration and participation are for everyone.

Why Does Getting Out Matter?

Being able to get around independently is crucial for:

- **Community Participation:** Transportation allows people to participate in activities, social events, and work opportunities within their communities.
- **Increased Independence:** The ability to travel independently boosts confidence and self-esteem.
- **Improved Quality of Life:** Exploring new places and connecting with others enriches our lives.

Using Public Transportation

Many public transportation systems offer accessibility features for people with disabilities. Here is what to consider:

- **Accessible Buses and Trains:** Look for features like ramps, designated seating areas, and audio announcements.
- **Trip Planning Resources:** Most public transportation systems offer online or phone-based trip planning tools with accessibility filters.
- **Paratransit Services:** Some areas offer specialized paratransit services for people who cannot use regular public transportation.

Adapted Vehicles and Transportation Options

For some people with disabilities, adapted vehicles might be necessary. Here are some options:

- **Handicap-accessible vans:** These vans have features like ramps, lowered floors, and hand controls for easier driving.
- **Vehicle modifications:** Cars can be modified with hand controls, swivel seats, or wheelchair lifts.
- **Ride-sharing services:** Some ride-sharing companies offer vehicles with accessibility features or partner with accessible transportation providers.

Travel Training and Route Planning

Planning your trip beforehand makes it smoother and less stressful. Here are some tips:

- **Practice Routes:** Familiarize yourself with routes and accessibility features beforehand, perhaps with a trusted companion.
- **Allow Extra Time:** Account for potential delays or unforeseen obstacles during your trip.
- **Learn to Use Public Transit Tools:** Understand how to purchase tickets, use maps, and navigate stations or stops.

Travel Assistance Services

There are services available to assist with travel if needed:

- **Personal Care Attendants (PCAs):** PCAs can provide assistance with boarding public transportation, navigating terminals, or carrying belongings.
- **Travel Training Programs:** These programs help individuals with disabilities learn to use public transportation independently.
- **Volunteer Escort Services:** Some organizations offer volunteer escorts to accompany individuals on their journeys.

Remember: Transportation and community access are essential for full participation in life. By exploring different options, planning your trips, and seeking assistance when needed, everyone can explore their communities and experience the joy of independent travel.

13. DENTAL HYGIENE

A healthy smile is more than just pearly whites. This chapter dives into the importance of oral care and brushing techniques for everyone, with a focus on helpful adaptations for people with disabilities.

Why Does a Healthy Mouth Matter?

Taking care of our teeth and gums is not just about a pretty smile. Oral health is linked to overall well-being:

- **Overall Health:** Poor oral hygiene can contribute to other health problems like heart disease or diabetes.
- **Pain and Discomfort:** Dental problems can be painful and interfere with eating and speaking.
- **Confidence Boost:** A healthy smile can boost self-confidence and overall well-being.

Brushing and Flossing Basics

Brushing and flossing are the cornerstones of good oral hygiene. Here is a breakdown:

- **Brushing:** Brush your teeth twice a day for two minutes each time. Use a soft-bristled toothbrush and fluoride toothpaste. Angle the brush at 45 degrees and brush gently in circular motions.

- **Flossing:** Floss daily to remove plaque and food particles between teeth. There are different flossing techniques, so find what works best for you.

Making Brushing Easier

For people with disabilities, there are tools and techniques that can make oral care easier. Here are some examples:

- **Electric toothbrushes:** These can be easier to use than manual toothbrushes, especially for people with limited hand function.
- **Flossing aids:** These tools can make flossing easier for people with dexterity challenges.
- **Thicker toothbrush handles:** These provide a better grip for people with limited hand strength.
- **Brushing with a partner or caregiver:** For some, assistance with brushing might be necessary.

Signs and Symptoms of Dental Problems

Regularly checking your mouth for signs of trouble can help prevent serious problems. Here is what to watch for:

- **Bleeding gums:** This can be a sign of gingivitis (gum inflammation).
- **Toothache or gum pain:** This can indicate a cavity, infection, or other dental problems.

- **Loose teeth:** Loose teeth can be a sign of gum disease.
- **Swollen gums:** This can be a sign of infection or other dental issues.

Importance of Regular Dental Visits

Regular dental checkups are crucial for maintaining good oral health. Here is why:

- **Early Detection:** A dentist can identify problems early on when they are easier and less expensive to treat.
- **Professional Cleaning:** Dentists can remove plaque and tartar buildup that brushing and flossing alone cannot reach.
- **Maintaining a Healthy Smile:** Regular checkups help ensure you keep your smile healthy and bright.

Remember: Oral hygiene is important for everyone, regardless of ability. By using proper brushing and flossing techniques, adapting routines when needed, and scheduling regular dental checkups, you can maintain a healthy mouth and a sparkling smile.

14. MANAGING CHRONIC CONDITIONS

Chronic conditions are health problems that require ongoing management. This chapter explores some common chronic conditions like diabetes, wound care, and respiratory care, empowering you to take an active role in your health. Remember, knowledge is power.

Understanding Chronic Conditions

Many chronic conditions exist, each requiring specific management strategies. Here is a brief overview of some common ones:

- **Diabetes:** A condition where the body struggles to regulate blood sugar levels. Management involves diet, exercise, and medication (if needed).
- **Wound Care:** Chronic wounds can take longer to heal. Proper cleaning, dressing changes, and infection prevention are crucial.
- **Respiratory Care:** Conditions like asthma or COPD (chronic obstructive pulmonary disease) can affect breathing. Techniques and devices can help manage these conditions.

Monitoring and Managing Diabetes

Diabetes requires close monitoring of blood sugar levels. Here is what you might need to do:

- **Blood Sugar Monitoring:** Use a glucometer to check your blood sugar regularly, following your doctor's instructions.
- **Healthy Eating:** A balanced diet helps control blood sugar.
- **Exercise:** Regular physical activity promotes healthy blood sugar levels.
- **Medications:** Some people with diabetes require medication to manage their blood sugar.

Techniques for Proper Wound Care

Chronic wounds need special attention to prevent infection and promote healing. Here are some key practices:

- **Wound Cleaning:** Clean the wound gently with prescribed solutions, following healthcare professional instructions.
- **Dressings:** Use appropriate dressings to keep the wound clean and protected.
- **Infection Prevention:** Practice good hand hygiene and watch for signs of infection like redness, swelling, or pus.

Respiratory Care Techniques and Assistive Devices

Certain conditions can make breathing difficult. Here are ways to manage these:

- **Breathing Techniques:** Techniques like pursed-lip breathing can help slow your breathing rate and ease discomfort.
- **Nebulizers:** These devices deliver medication in a mist inhaled through a mask or mouthpiece to open airways.
- **CPAP Machines:** These machines use continuous positive airway pressure to keep airways open during sleep for some conditions.

Working Together with Healthcare Professionals

Chronic condition management is a team effort. Here is how to collaborate with your healthcare providers:

- **Regular Checkups:** Attend scheduled appointments to monitor your condition and adjust treatment plans if needed.
- **Ask Questions:** Do not hesitate to ask questions and voice any concerns you have.
- **Follow Instructions:** Carefully follow your healthcare professional's recommendations for medication, diet, and other management strategies.

Remember: Chronic conditions do not have to define you. By understanding your condition, taking an active role in your management, and working with your healthcare team, you can live a healthy and fulfilling life. Always consult your healthcare professional for personalized guidance on managing your specific chronic condition.

15. SEIZURE CARE

Seizures are sudden surges of electrical activity in the brain that can cause temporary changes in behavior, sensation, or awareness. This chapter equips caregivers, family members, and anyone interacting with individuals with epilepsy with the knowledge and skills to provide support and ensure safety during seizures.

Understanding Different Seizures and Triggers

Epilepsy manifests in various seizure types, each with distinct characteristics. Here is a basic breakdown:

- **Focal Seizures:** These affect a specific part of the brain, causing localized symptoms like twitching in a limb or changes in sensation.
- **Generalized Seizures:** These involve the entire brain, causing loss of consciousness, body stiffening, or jerking movements.
- **Absence Seizures:** These brief seizures involve short periods of blank staring or daydreaming, often going unnoticed by others.

Some individuals experience warning signs, called auras, before a seizure. These can include unusual smells, tastes, or feelings of déjà vu. Identifying potential triggers, like stress or lack of sleep, can also help individuals with epilepsy manage their condition.

Recognizing Impending Seizures

Being aware of potential seizure warnings can make a big difference in ensuring safety. Here is what to watch for:

- **Auras:** Unusual sensations, smells, or tastes may precede a seizure.
- **Behavioral Changes:** Sudden confusion, restlessness, or withdrawal might indicate an impending seizure.
- **Physical Changes:** Rapid blinking, muscle twitching, or changes in breathing patterns could be warning signs.

Creating a Safe Environment

A safe environment minimizes the risk of injury during a seizure. Here are some tips:

- **Remove Obstacles:** Clear the area around the person of furniture or sharp objects to prevent falls or injuries.
- **Pad the Floor:** If possible, place a pillow or blanket underneath the person to cushion any potential fall.
- **Stay Calm:** Although witnessing a seizure can be alarming, stay calm and speak in a reassuring tone.

First Aid Procedures During Seizures

During a seizure, the primary goal is to ensure safety and avoid interference with the natural course of the seizure. Here is what to do:

- **Do not Restrain:** Do not attempt to restrain the person during a seizure. This can cause injuries.
- **Gently Guide:** If the person is in danger of falling, gently guide them to a safe position on the floor.
- **Clear the Mouth:** Remove any objects from the person's mouth to prevent choking, but do not force anything open.
- **Time the Seizure:** Keep track of the seizure duration using a watch or phone. Seizures lasting longer than five minutes require immediate medical attention.

Post-Seizure Care and Support

Once the seizure subsides, focus on comfort and support. Here is how to help:

- **Stay with the Person:** Remain with the person until they regain full awareness and can communicate clearly.
- **Offer Comfort:** Speak in a calm and reassuring tone. Offer assistance if needed, such as helping them sit up or get a drink of water.

- **Respect Privacy:** If the person needs time to recover privately, offer them space.

Remember: Epilepsy is a manageable condition. By understanding different seizure types, recognizing warning signs, creating a safe environment, and knowing basic first aid procedures, you can effectively support individuals with epilepsy and ensure their well-being. Always consult a healthcare professional for personalized guidance on managing epilepsy and seizure care.

16. HOME HEALTHCARE TEAM

Home healthcare allows individuals with disabilities or needing recovery to receive care in the comfort of their own homes. This chapter explores the different types of home healthcare professionals, their roles, and how to build effective communication for optimal care. Remember, a strong team approach leads to better health outcomes.

Different Types of Healthcare Professionals

A variety of skilled professionals can be part of a home healthcare team, each with specialized expertise. Here is a look at some key players:

- **Registered Nurses (RNs):** RNs provide a wide range of services, including medication management, wound care, patient education, and monitoring vital signs.
- **Physical Therapists (PTs):** PTs help individuals regain strength, mobility, and improve functional abilities for daily living tasks.
- **Occupational Therapists (OTs):** OTs focus on helping people regain independence in performing daily activities like dressing, bathing, and self-care tasks.
- **Speech-Language Pathologists (SLPs):** SLPs work with people experiencing difficulty with communication, swallowing, or cognitive function.

- **Home Health Support Aides:** Aides provide assistance with daily activities like bathing, dressing, meal preparation, and light housekeeping.

Understanding Their Expertise

Each home healthcare professional brings unique skills to the table. Here is a simplified breakdown of their roles:

- **Nurses:** They assess health needs, administer medications, monitor progress, and coordinate care with doctors.
- **Physical Therapists:** They create exercise programs to improve strength, balance, and movement capabilities.
- **Occupational Therapists:** They teach adaptive techniques for performing daily activities and maximizing independence.
- **Speech-Language Pathologists:** They help improve communication skills, swallowing difficulties, and cognitive function.
- **Home Health Aides:** They provide physical assistance with daily living tasks, promoting independence and well-being.

Effective Communication

Open communication is crucial for successful home healthcare. Here is how to build strong relationships with your care team:

- **Ask Questions:** Do not hesitate to ask questions about your care plan, procedures, or medications.
- **Express Concerns:** Voice any concerns you might have regarding your health or the care being provided.
- **Provide Information:** Share any relevant medical history, symptoms, or changes in your condition.

Coordinating Care Plans and Sharing Information

A coordinated care plan ensures everyone on the team is on the same page. Here is how to ensure smooth communication:

- **Care Plan Meetings:** Attend meetings with your healthcare team to discuss the plan, goals, and progress.
- **Sharing Information:** Share information about doctor's appointments, medications, or any changes with all team members.
- **Joint Communication:** Encourage communication between your home healthcare team and your doctor to ensure seamless care.

Advocating for the Needs of the Individual

You, or the individual receiving care, are an essential part of the team. Here is how to advocate for your needs:

- **Be Clear About Your Goals:** Communicate your desired outcomes and what's important in your care.
- **Make Informed Decisions:** Ask questions and understand your treatment options before making choices.
- **Express Preferences:** Voice your preferences for care delivery and communication style.

Remember: A strong home healthcare team can significantly improve quality of life. By understanding the roles of each professional, communicating effectively, and advocating for your needs, you can create a collaborative environment that fosters optimal health and well-being.

17. CARING FOR PHYSICAL DISABILITIES

Physical disabilities encompass a wide range of conditions affecting movement, strength, and coordination. This chapter explores various disabilities, their impact on daily life, and strategies for providing compassionate and effective care. Remember, a little support goes a long way in promoting well-being and independence.

Types of Physical Disabilities

Physical disabilities manifest in many forms, each with unique challenges. Here is a brief overview of some common types:

- **Spinal Cord Injuries (SCIs):** SCIs can affect movement, sensation, and bladder/bowel control depending on the injury level.
- **Amputations:** Loss of limbs can impact mobility and require prosthetic devices and adaptation for daily activities.
- **Muscular Dystrophy:** A group of muscle diseases causing progressive weakness and affecting movement and independence.
- **Cerebral Palsy:** A condition affecting movement, coordination, and speech due to brain development issues.

Each disability has its own set of challenges, impacting

daily activities like bathing, dressing, mobility, and self-care.

Specific Care Needs for Different Disabilities

The specific care needs of individuals with physical disabilities vary depending on the type and severity of their condition. Here are some general considerations:

- **Mobility Assistance:** People with mobility limitations may require wheelchairs, walkers, or other assistive devices to move around safely.
- **Transferring and Positioning:** Assistance might be needed with transferring from bed to chair, toileting, or maintaining proper positioning to prevent pressure sores.
- **Daily Living Activities:** Support may be needed with bathing, dressing, eating, grooming, and other daily tasks.
- **Adaptive Equipment:** Specialized equipment like grab bars, raised toilet seats, or long-handled tools can promote independence.

Pain Management Strategies

Chronic pain is a common challenge for people with physical disabilities. Here are some strategies for managing pain:

- **Medication:** Pain medication prescribed by a doctor can help manage pain levels.
- **Physical Therapy:** Exercises can strengthen muscles, improve flexibility, and reduce pain.
- **Heat or Cold Therapy:** Applying heat or cold packs to affected areas can provide temporary pain relief.
- **Relaxation Techniques:** Meditation, deep breathing exercises, and stress management can help manage pain perception.

Importance of Exercise and Physical Therapy

Maintaining physical activity is crucial for overall health and well-being for individuals with physical disabilities. Here is why:

- **Improved Mobility:** Exercise strengthens muscles, improves balance, and can increase functional capacity.
- **Reduced Pain:** Physical activity can help manage chronic pain and improve overall fitness.
- **Psychological Benefits:** Exercise can boost mood, reduce stress, and promote a sense of well-being.

Physical therapy programs can be customized to address individual needs and limitations, promoting safe and effective exercise routines.

Psychological Considerations

Living with a physical disability can have a significant emotional impact. Here is what to consider:

- **Counseling:** Therapy can help individuals cope with adjustment, anxiety, or depression related to their disability.
- **Support Groups:** Connecting with others facing similar challenges can provide emotional support and a sense of community.
- **Positive Reinforcement:** Celebrating accomplishments and focusing on strengths can boost self-esteem and motivation.

Remember: Providing care for individuals with physical disabilities is a journey of compassion and collaboration. By understanding the specific needs of each situation, offering tailored support, and promoting physical and emotional well-being, we can empower individuals with disabilities to live fulfilling and independent lives.

18. VISION AND HEARING IMPAIRMENTS

The world is a symphony of sights and sounds. This chapter explores different types of vision and hearing impairments, along with communication strategies and assistive devices that can bridge the sensory gap and empower individuals to connect and participate fully in life. Remember, a little understanding goes a long way in building a more inclusive world.

Understanding Vision Impairments

Vision impairments range from complete blindness to varying degrees of low vision. Here is a basic breakdown:

- **Blindness:** Complete or near-complete loss of sight.
- **Low Vision:** Partially impaired vision that cannot be corrected with glasses or contact lenses.

Individuals with low vision might experience blurred vision, tunnel vision, or difficulty seeing in low light.

Communication Strategies for Vision Impairments

Effective communication is essential. Here are some strategies to interact with individuals who are blind or visually impaired:

- **Identify Yourself:** Always announce yourself when entering a room or approaching someone.
- **Speak Clearly:** Speak at a normal pace and volume, and avoid mumbling.
- **Describe Your Surroundings:** If guiding someone, verbally describe the environment, including obstacles or changes in direction.
- **Braille:** Learn basic Braille phrases like "hello" or "excuse me" to show respect and awareness.
- **Audio Descriptions:** Utilize audio descriptions for movies, videos, or presentations that provide a narrated description of visual elements.

Assistive Devices for Vision Impairments

Many assistive devices can enhance independence for people with vision impairments. Here are a few examples:

- **White Canes:** These canes help navigate surroundings by detecting obstacles.
- **Guide Dogs:** Specially trained dogs assist with mobility and provide companionship.
- **Magnifiers:** These devices enlarge printed materials for easier reading.
- **Text-to-Speech Software:** This software converts digital text into spoken words for computers and smartphones.

Different Types of Hearing Impairments

Hearing impairments can range from mild to complete deafness. Here is a basic breakdown:

- **Deafness:** Complete or near-complete loss of hearing.
- **Hard of Hearing:** Partially impaired hearing, where sounds might be muffled, faint, or difficult to understand.

Communication Strategies for Hearing Impairments

Clear communication is key. Here is how to interact effectively with individuals who are deaf or hard of hearing:

- **Get Attention:** Make eye contact or wave to gain their attention before speaking.
- **Face the Person:** Speaking directly allows them to see your facial expressions and lip movements.
- **Speak Clearly:** Articulate words clearly, but avoid shouting.
- **Use Sign Language:** Learn basic signs or gestures for common phrases to enhance communication.
- **Assistive Listening Devices:** Utilize devices like amplified phones or FM systems that improve sound clarity.

Assistive Devices for Hearing Impairments

Technology plays a crucial role in assisting individuals with hearing loss. Here are some examples:

- **Hearing Aids:** Electronic devices that amplify sounds and improve hearing ability.
- **Alerting Systems:** Devices that use flashing lights or vibrations to alert individuals to sounds like doorbells or alarms.
- **Closed Captioning:** Text captions displayed on screens that correspond to spoken dialogue in videos or television shows.

Remember: Vision and hearing impairments are not limitations. By understanding these conditions, utilizing communication strategies, and incorporating assistive devices, we can create a more inclusive environment where everyone can participate and thrive.

19. INTELLECTUAL AND DEVELOPMENTAL DISABILITIES

Intellectual and developmental disabilities (ID/DD) encompass a wide range of conditions affecting cognitive development and functioning. This chapter explores different types of ID/DD, common challenges, and positive strategies to promote communication, independence, and a fulfilling life. Remember, every individual is unique, and understanding their needs is key to building a supportive environment.

Types of Intellectual and Developmental Disabilities

ID/DD refers to a group of conditions with varying degrees of severity. Here are some common examples:

- **Down Syndrome:** A genetic condition causing intellectual disability and distinct physical features.
- **Autism Spectrum Disorder (ASD):** A developmental condition characterized by social communication challenges and restricted interests.
- **Intellectual Disability (ID):** A general term for significant limitations in cognitive skills that impact daily life.

Characteristics and Challenges

Individuals with ID/DD may experience various challenges, depending on the specific condition. Some common characteristics include:

- **Difficulties with Communication:** Limited verbal skills, trouble understanding complex language, or challenges with social interaction.
- **Learning Delays:** Difficulties with academics, problem solving, or following instructions.
- **Developmental Delays:** Slow development of motor skills, social skills, or self-care skills.

Positive Behavioral Support Strategies

Positive behavioral support focuses on identifying and addressing triggers for challenging behaviors. Here are some key strategies:

- **Identify Triggers:** Understand what situations or environments might lead to behavioral issues.
- **Provide Clear Routines:** Establish predictable routines and schedules to create a sense of security.
- **Positive Reinforcement:** Reward desired behaviors with praise, encouragements, or preferred activities.
- **Visual Aids:** Use pictures, charts, or other visual supports to communicate expectations and instructions.

- **Calm De-escalation Techniques:** Learn techniques to de-escalate stressful situations without confrontation.

Communication Techniques

Effective communication is crucial for building relationships and promoting independence. Here are some tips for interacting with individuals with ID/DD:

- **Use Simple Language:** Speak slowly and clearly, using short sentences and concrete words.
- **Focus on Nonverbal Cues:** Pay attention to facial expressions and body language to understand their needs.
- **Offer Choices:** Present options in a simple way to encourage participation and decision-making.
- **Be Patient:** Allow extra time for understanding and processing information.
- **Visual Aids:** Pictures, gestures, and demonstrations can complement verbal communication.

Promoting Skill Development

Encouraging skill development fosters a sense of accomplishment and independence. Here is how to support individuals with ID/DD:

- **Break Down Tasks:** Divide tasks into smaller, manageable steps with clear instructions.
- **Practice Makes Progress:** Provide opportunities for repetition and practice to develop skills.
- **Celebrate Achievements:** Recognize and celebrate improvements, no matter how small.
- **Focus on Strengths:** Build on individual strengths and interests to promote motivation and self-confidence.
- **Promote Self-Advocacy:** Encourage individuals to communicate their needs and preferences as they develop communication skills.

Remember: Intellectual and developmental disabilities are not defining characteristics. By understanding individual needs, utilizing positive support strategies, and promoting communication and skill development, we can empower individuals with ID/DD to live fulfilling and independent lives. Always consult with healthcare professionals and qualified support staff for personalized guidance on supporting individuals with specific ID/DD diagnoses.

20. SUPPORTING MENTAL WELLBEING

Mental health is an essential part of overall well-being. This chapter explores common mental health conditions, their signs and symptoms, and strategies for supporting individuals experiencing emotional challenges. Remember, mental health conditions are treatable, and seeking help is a sign of strength.

Common Mental Health Conditions

Many mental health conditions exist, each with unique characteristics. Here is a brief overview of some common ones:

- **Anxiety Disorders:** Excessive worry, fear, and physical symptoms like rapid heart rate or difficulty breathing.
- **Depression:** Persistent feelings of sadness, hopelessness, and loss of interest in activities.
- **Bipolar Disorder:** Mood swings between extreme highs (mania) and lows (depression).
- **Eating Disorders:** Unhealthy eating habits and distorted body image.
- **Post-Traumatic Stress Disorder (PTSD):** Symptoms like flashbacks, nightmares, and avoidance after a traumatic event.

Recognizing the Signs and Symptoms

Mental health conditions can manifest in various ways. Here are some general signs to watch for:

- **Changes in Mood:** Persistent sadness, irritability, mania, or anxiety.
- **Changes in Behavior:** Social withdrawal, changes in sleep or eating patterns, increased substance use.
- **Changes in Thinking:** Difficulty concentrating, negative thoughts about oneself or the future.
- **Physical Symptoms:** Fatigue, headaches, stomachaches, or changes in appetite.

Offering a Safe Space

If someone you know is struggling, here is how to offer support:

- **Listen Without Judgment:** Create a safe space for them to express their feelings without judgment.
- **Offer Encouragement:** Let them know you care and believe in their ability to feel better.
- **Help Them Seek Help:** Encourage them to talk to a doctor or mental health professional.
- **Offer Practical Support:** Help them with daily tasks or accompany them to appointments.

Crisis Intervention and De-escalation Techniques

In times of crisis, here are some steps to take:

- **Stay Calm:** Your calmness can help de-escalate the situation.
- **Active Listening:** Listen attentively and validate their feelings.
- **Speak Calmly and Clearly:** Avoid yelling or arguing.
- **Remove Harmful Objects:** If there is a risk of self-harm, remove any harmful objects from the environment.
- **Encourage Professional Help:** Call emergency services or a mental health crisis hotline if needed.

Medication Adherence and Therapy

Treatment for mental health conditions often involves a combination of medication and therapy. Here is why both are important:

- **Medication:** Medications can help manage symptoms like anxiety, depression, or mood swings.
- **Therapy:** Therapy provides tools for coping with emotional challenges, developing healthy coping mechanisms, and building resilience.

- **Adherence is Key:** Taking medication as prescribed by a doctor is crucial for optimal treatment outcomes.

Remember: Mental health conditions are not a sign of weakness. With support, proper treatment, and self-care, individuals can manage their mental health and live fulfilling lives. If you are experiencing mental health challenges, know that help is available. You are not alone.

21. LEARNING DISABILITIES

Learning disabilities (LD) are a group of neurodevelopmental conditions that can affect how a person processes and interprets information. This chapter explores different types of LDs, the challenges they present, and strategies for promoting effective learning and organization skills. Remember, with the right support and tools, individuals with LDs can achieve their full potential.

Types of Learning Disabilities

Learning disabilities manifest in various ways, each impacting specific areas of learning. Here are some common types:

- **Dyslexia:** Difficulty with reading, including problems with accuracy, fluency, and comprehension.
- **Dysgraphia:** Challenges with written expression, affecting spelling, handwriting, and fine motor skills.
- **Dyscalculia:** Difficulties with math concepts, including understanding numbers, performing calculations, and solving problems.
- **Attention Deficit Hyperactivity Disorder (ADHD):** While not exclusively a learning disability, ADHD can significantly impact focus,

attention, and organization, affecting learning processes.

Challenges of Learning Disabilities

Individuals with LDs might experience challenges in various aspects of daily life. Here are some common ones:

- **Academic Difficulties:** Struggling with reading, writing, math, or following instructions can hinder academic progress.
- **Low Self-Esteem:** Challenges with learning can lead to frustration and feelings of inadequacy.
- **Organization Problems:** Difficulties with planning, time management, and keeping track of assignments can impact overall functioning.
- **Social Challenges:** Learning differences can sometimes lead to social isolation or misunderstandings.

Learning Strategies and Assistive Technologies

There are many strategies and tools to empower individuals with LDs. Here are a few examples:

- **Learning Strategies:** Techniques like breaking down instructions, using graphic organizers, or employing mnemonic devices can enhance understanding and retention.

- **Assistive Technologies:** Text-to-speech software, audiobooks, spellcheckers, or voice recorders can provide valuable support for reading, writing, and organization.
- **Structured Learning Environments:** Clear routines, predictable schedules, and consistent expectations can create a stable and supportive learning environment.

Promoting Organization and Time Management Skills

Developing strong organizational skills is crucial for individuals with LDs. Here are some ways to help:

- **Visual Aids:** Utilize calendars, planners, checklists, or color-coding systems to keep track of tasks and deadlines.
- **Chunking Information:** Break down large projects or assignments into smaller, more manageable steps.
- **Time Management Techniques:** Set realistic deadlines, use timers, and prioritize tasks to stay on track.
- **Develop Routines:** Establish consistent routines for completing homework, studying, and other daily activities.

Advocating for Accommodations

Individuals with LDs may need accommodations in educational and work settings to ensure equal access to opportunities. Here is how to advocate for support:

- **Know Your Rights:** Learn about disability laws and accommodations available in educational and work environments.
- **Communicate Needs:** Openly discuss learning disabilities with teachers, professors, or employers.
- **Develop a Support Plan:** Work collaboratively with educators or employers to create a plan outlining specific accommodations, such as extended time on tests, note-taking assistance, or modified assignments.

Remember: Learning disabilities are not a reflection of intelligence. With the right support, effective learning strategies, and access to appropriate accommodations, individuals with LDs can achieve academic success, thrive in their careers, and lead fulfilling lives.

22. AUTISM SPECTRUM DISORDER

Autism Spectrum Disorder (ASD) is a developmental condition characterized by social communication challenges and restricted interests. This chapter explores the core characteristics of ASD, strategies for understanding and responding to challenging behaviors, and methods to promote effective communication, social skills development, and sensory processing accommodation. Remember, every individual on the spectrum is unique, and understanding their specific needs is key to providing effective support.

Core Characteristics of ASD

ASD manifests in a variety of ways, but some core characteristics are common across the spectrum. Here is a breakdown of some key aspects:

- **Social Communication Challenges:** Difficulties with understanding nonverbal cues, initiating conversations, and maintaining eye contact.
- **Restricted Interests:** Intense focus on specific topics or activities, often accompanied by repetitive behaviors.
- **Sensory Processing Issues:** Over- or under-sensitivity to sights, sounds, textures, tastes, or smells.

These core characteristics can lead to challenges in various aspects of life, including communication, social interaction, and navigating daily routines.

Challenging Behaviors

Individuals with ASD might exhibit challenging behaviors like tantrums, meltdowns, or repetitive movements. These behaviors are often a way of communicating distress or needs. Here is how to approach them:

- **Identify Triggers:** Try to understand what situations or sensory stimuli might be triggering the behavior.
- **Stay Calm and De-escalate:** Maintaining a calm presence can help de-escalate the situation.
- **Provide Clear Communication:** Use simple language and visual cues to communicate expectations.
- **Create a Safe Space:** If needed, provide a quiet space for the individual to calm down.
- **Seek Professional Guidance:** Consult with therapists specializing in ASD behavior management for tailored strategies.

Effective Communication Strategies

Communication is essential for building relationships and reducing frustration. Here are some tips for communicating effectively with individuals with ASD:

- **Use Simple and Direct Language:** Avoid idioms, sarcasm, or figurative speech that can be confusing.
- **Focus on Visual Communication:** Utilize pictures, charts, or written instructions to support verbal communication.
- **Respect Personal Space:** Be mindful of potential sensitivities to touch or proximity.
- **Allow Processing Time:** Individuals with ASD may need extra time to understand information and respond.
- **Focus on Interests:** Use their interests as a starting point to engage them in conversation.

Social Skills Training and Development

Social interactions can be challenging for individuals with ASD. Social skills training can help them develop tools for:

- **Understanding Social Cues:** Learn to interpret body language, facial expressions, and social norms.
- **Initiating and Maintaining Conversations:** Practice starting and keeping conversations going with others.
- **Nonverbal Communication:** Develop skills like making eye contact and using appropriate gestures.

- **Building Relationships:** Learn how to build friendships and navigate social interactions.

Sensory Processing Issues and Strategies for Accommodation

Individuals with ASD may experience sensory input differently. Here is how to create a more comfortable environment:

- **Identify Sensory Sensitivities:** Pay attention to what sights, sounds, textures, or smells might be overwhelming.
- **Offer Sensory Outlets:** Provide fidget toys, noise-cancelling headphones, or calming activities for sensory regulation.
- **Create Predictable Routines:** Establish predictable routines and schedules that provide a sense of security.
- **Offer Choices:** When possible, offer choices related to sensory experiences, like clothing or lighting.
- **Calm Down Techniques:** Teach calming techniques like deep breathing or taking breaks to manage sensory overload.

Remember: ASD is a spectrum, and every individual experiences it differently. With understanding, effective communication strategies, and support for social skills development and sensory needs, individuals with ASD can thrive and connect with the world around them.

23. SUPPORTING INDIVIDUALS WHO USE SIGN LANGUAGE AND ASSISTIVE DEVICES

The world of communication is vast and varied. This chapter delves deeper into the specific needs of individuals who use sign language due to deafness or hearing loss. We will explore considerations for caregivers, delve into Deaf culture and etiquette, and revisit assistive technologies that can enhance daily living. Remember, effective communication is a two-way street, and a little understanding goes a long way in building strong relationships.

Understanding Sign Language Users

While some individuals with deafness or hearing loss may rely on spoken language with the help of hearing aids or speech therapy, others utilize sign language as their primary mode of communication. Here is what caregivers should consider:

- **Learn Basic Signs:** Start with simple greetings, essential phrases, and signs related to daily activities. Many online resources and classes can help with basic sign language acquisition.
- **Respect Sign Language Space:** Maintain a clear view of the person's face and hands while signing. Avoid interrupting or standing too close.

- **Get Attention Before Speaking:** A gentle tap on the shoulder or waving your hand can effectively gain attention without being startling.
- **Be Patient:** Sign language is a complex language with its own grammar and syntax. Allow time for processing and communication.
- **Utilize Additional Supports:** Written notes, pictures, or pointing can supplement sign language communication, especially in complex situations.

Embracing a Culture: Deaf Culture and Etiquette

Deafness is not just a disability; it is also a cultural identity with its own rich history, traditions, and values. Here are some important points of Deaf culture etiquette:

- **Deafness is not a disability in Deaf culture.** It is a different way of experiencing the world.
- **Signing is a complete and natural language.** It is not simply a way to represent spoken language.
- **Maintain eye contact while signing.** This demonstrates attentiveness and respect in Deaf culture.
- **Use a sign language interpreter** in formal settings where clear communication is crucial.
- **Be inclusive.** Deaf individuals enrich our communities. Embrace opportunities to learn and celebrate Deaf culture.

Assistive Technologies for Daily Living

Technology plays a vital role in supporting individuals with deafness or hearing loss. Here is a look at some helpful devices:

- **Alerting Systems:** Light flashes, vibrating devices, or bed shakers can alert individuals to doorbells, alarms, or smoke detectors.
- **Captioning and Transcription Services:** Real-time captioning on televisions, phones, or video conferencing platforms can improve communication access.
- **Amplified Phones:** These phones increase the volume of incoming calls, making conversations easier to understand.
- **Hearing Aids:** Electronic devices that amplify sounds and improve hearing ability, especially for individuals with some residual hearing.

Remember: Communication is a cornerstone of human connection. By respecting Deaf culture, learning basic signs, and utilizing assistive technologies, we can create a more inclusive environment where everyone can participate and thrive.

24. VISUAL IMPAIRMENTS

The world is a tapestry of sights, but for individuals with visual impairments, experiencing their surroundings requires a different approach. This chapter explores ways to create accessible environments, the benefits of assistive technologies, and techniques for safe and independent travel. Remember, a few modifications can open doors to a world of possibilities.

Environmental Modifications for the Home

Our homes are our sanctuaries. Here are some ways to modify living spaces for increased accessibility for individuals with visual impairments:

- **Lighting:** Ensure adequate and even lighting throughout the home. Avoid harsh contrasts and use dimmer switches for adjustability.
- **Color Contrast:** Utilize contrasting colors for walls, floors, and furniture to create clear boundaries and define spaces.
- **Clear Pathways:** Maintain clear walkways free of clutter to prevent tripping hazards.
- **Tactile Cues:** Place textured strips on stairs or bathroom floors to warn of changes in elevation.
- **Labeling:** Use braille labels or large print labels on appliances, cabinets, and storage containers for easy identification.

Assistive Technologies for Daily Living

Technology plays a crucial role in promoting independence for individuals with visual impairments. Here are some helpful devices:

- **Talking Devices:** These devices announce information electronically, such as talking clocks, watches, or thermometers.
- **Screen Readers:** Software programs that convert digital text on computers or smartphones into spoken instructions, allowing individuals to access information independently.
- **Magnifiers:** Handheld or electronic devices that enlarge printed materials for easier reading.
- **Optical Character Recognition (OCR) Software:** This software converts printed text into digital text, allowing individuals to access information on documents or images through a screen reader.
- **Assistive Navigation Devices:** Electronic canes or personal navigation devices can provide audio cues and guidance for safe travel.

Travel Techniques and Orientation

Traveling independently can be empowering. Here are some strategies to support individuals with visual impairments when navigating their surroundings:

- **Orientation and Mobility Training:** Programs teach individuals safe travel techniques, using canes or guide dogs, and developing mental maps of familiar environments.
- **Public Transportation Accessibility:** Many public transportation systems offer features like audio announcements or tactile guidance strips to assist visually impaired passengers.
- **Descriptive Services for Travel:** Apps or services provide detailed audio descriptions of landmarks or locations, enhancing the travel experience.
- **Planning and Preparation:** Researching routes, identifying landmarks, and requesting assistance when needed can contribute to a smooth travel experience.

Remember: Visual impairments do not limit potential. By creating accessible environments, utilizing assistive technologies, and promoting travel skills, we can empower individuals with visual impairments to explore the world with confidence and independence.

25. CREATING AN ACCESSIBLE HOME ENVIRONMENT

Our homes are our sanctuaries, and ensuring they are accessible benefits everyone, not just individuals with disabilities. This chapter explores home accessibility assessments, various adaptive equipment options, and universal design principles. By incorporating these elements, we can create a safe and comfortable living environment for all.

Home Accessibility Assessments and Modifications

The first step is to assess your current living space. Here are some considerations:

- **Accessibility Professionals:** Occupational therapists or certified accessibility specialists can conduct a home assessment to identify areas needing modification.
- **Individual Needs:** Consider the specific needs of residents, whether mobility limitations, visual impairments, or hearing difficulties.
- **Prioritizing Modifications:** Focus on high-impact modifications that significantly improve accessibility in essential areas like bathrooms, kitchens, and entryways.

Adaptive Equipment for Daily Living

A variety of adaptive equipment can enhance independence in daily activities. Here are some examples:

- **Bathroom Safety:** Grab bars around the shower, bathtub, and toilet can provide stability and prevent falls. Raised toilet seats can also improve accessibility.
- **Kitchen Modifications:** Lower cabinets for easier reach, stovetop controls at an accessible height, and lever-handled faucets are some helpful adaptations.
- **Doorways and Entrances:** Widening doorways to accommodate wheelchairs or walkers and installing ramps over thresholds can improve ease of movement.
- **Lighting and Contrast:** Adequate lighting throughout the home, along with contrasting colors for walls, floors, and furniture, can enhance visibility for those with visual impairments.

Universal Design Principles for Creating an Accessible Home

Universal Design (UD) focuses on creating spaces usable by everyone, regardless of ability. Here are some core UD principles:

- **Equitable Use:** The design should be usable by people with diverse abilities.
- **Flexibility:** The space should adapt to different needs and preferences.
- **Simple and Intuitive Use:** Features should be easy to understand and operate.
- **Perceptible Information:** Information should be communicated effectively through visual, auditory, or tactile means.
- **Low Physical Effort:** Minimize the physical effort required to use the space and its features.
- **Size and Space for Approach and Use:** Provide sufficient space for maneuvering wheelchairs, walkers, or other mobility aids.

Safety Considerations for Individuals with Disabilities in the Home

Safety is paramount. Here are some additional considerations:

- **Fall Prevention:** Install grab bars in bathrooms, remove loose rugs, and ensure proper lighting to minimize fall risks.
- **Fire Safety:** Install smoke detectors and carbon monoxide detectors throughout the home and ensure they are functioning properly.
- **Electrical Safety:** Cover unused outlets and consider installing GFCI outlets in bathrooms and kitchens.

- **Emergency Communication:** Have a plan for emergency communication, such as a readily accessible phone or medical alert system.

Remember: An accessible home environment fosters independence, dignity, and a sense of security for everyone. By conducting assessments, incorporating adaptive equipment, and embracing universal design principles, we can create homes that embrace and celebrate diversity.

26. BUILDING A SUPPORT NETWORK

Living with a disability or caring for someone with a disability does not have to be a solitary journey. This chapter explores the wealth of resources available in the community, the benefits of support groups, and the importance of advocacy and collaboration. Together, we can build a more inclusive and supportive environment.

Identifying Relevant Community Resources

Numerous community resources exist to assist individuals with disabilities and their caregivers. Here is how to navigate these resources:

- **Disability Organizations:** National and local organizations focused on specific disabilities offer information, support programs, and advocacy efforts.
- **Government Agencies:** Many government agencies provide resources and services for individuals with disabilities, such as vocational rehabilitation, housing assistance, or financial aid programs.
- **Support Groups:** Connecting with others facing similar challenges can be incredibly helpful. Support groups offer emotional support, shared experiences, and valuable information.

- **Transportation Services:** Accessible transportation options like paratransit services can help individuals with mobility limitations maintain independence.
- **Assistive Technology Resources:** Organizations or agencies may offer assistance in identifying, acquiring, or learning to use assistive technology.

Benefits of Participating in Support Groups

Support groups offer a unique space for individuals with disabilities and caregivers to connect and share experiences. Here are some of the benefits of participation:

- **Emotional Support:** Feeling understood and supported by others facing similar challenges can be a tremendous source of strength and encouragement.
- **Information Sharing:** Learning from others' experiences, successes, and strategies can be invaluable in managing daily life.
- **Sense of Community:** Building friendships and connections can combat feelings of isolation and empower individuals to advocate for themselves.
- **Caregiver Support:** Support groups specifically for caregivers provide a safe space to share concerns, learn coping mechanisms, and access resources for managing their own well-being.

Advocacy and Collaboration with Community Organizations

Advocacy involves speaking up for the rights and needs of individuals with disabilities. Here is how to get involved:

- **Connect with Disability Advocacy Groups:** These organizations work to shape policies and legislation promoting inclusion and accessibility.
- **Educate Others:** Raise awareness about specific disabilities and challenge misconceptions.
- **Support Inclusive Initiatives:** Advocate for accessible public spaces, transportation options, and educational opportunities.
- **Work with Community Organizations:** Collaborate with local organizations to create a more inclusive and supportive community for everyone.

Remember: Building a supportive network is crucial. By utilizing community resources, participating in support groups, and engaging in advocacy efforts, we can create a world where everyone has the opportunity to thrive. Together, we can make a difference.

27. SELF-CARE FOR CAREGIVERS

The role of a caregiver is demanding and rewarding in equal measure. However, neglecting your own well-being can lead to burnout, hindering your ability to care for yourself and others effectively. This chapter emphasizes the importance of self-care for caregivers and explores strategies for managing stress, maintaining emotional well-being, and prioritizing your physical health. Remember, a well-rested and healthy caregiver is a better caregiver.

Why Self-Care Matters

Caregiving can be emotionally and physically draining. Constant stress can lead to burnout, characterized by exhaustion, cynicism, and a reduced sense of accomplishment. Self-care is not a luxury; it is essential for preventing burnout and ensuring you can continue to provide quality care.

Managing Stress and Maintaining Emotional Wellbeing

Here are some strategies to combat stress and nurture your emotional well-being:

- **Identify Stressors:** Recognize situations or triggers that cause you stress.

- **Relaxation Techniques:** Practice relaxation techniques like deep breathing, meditation, or progressive muscle relaxation to manage stress in the moment.
- **Maintain Positive Outlets:** Engage in activities you enjoy, whether it is reading, spending time in nature, or connecting with loved ones.
- **Set Realistic Expectations:** Do not try to be superhuman. Accept that you cannot do everything perfectly and delegate tasks when possible.
- **Seek Professional Help:** If stress feels overwhelming, consider therapy or counseling for support and coping mechanisms.

Prioritization for Caregivers

Time management is crucial for caregivers. Here are some tips to juggle your responsibilities:

- **Create a Schedule:** Plan your days and weeks, including time for caregiving tasks, self-care activities, and personal needs.
- **Prioritize ruthlessly:** Focus on the most important tasks first and delegate or reschedule less urgent ones.
- **Learn to Say No:** It is okay to set boundaries and decline additional commitments if you are feeling overloaded.

- **Ask for Help:** Do not be afraid to ask family, friends, or community services for help with errands, transportation, or respite care.

Importance of Physical Health

Taking care of your physical health directly impacts your emotional well-being. Here is how to prioritize your physical health:

- **Healthy Eating:** Fuel your body with nutritious foods to maintain energy levels and overall health.
- **Regular Exercise:** Physical activity is a natural stress reliever and mood booster. Aim for at least 30 minutes of moderate-intensity exercise most days of the week.
- **Adequate Sleep:** Aim for 7-8 hours of quality sleep each night to feel refreshed and energized.

Building Your Support System

You do not have to go through this alone. Here are ways to build your support system:

- **Connect with Other Caregivers:** Support groups can provide a safe space to share experiences, find understanding, and gain emotional support.

- **Talk to Friends and Family:** Lean on your loved ones for emotional support and practical help.
- **Seek Professional Help:** Therapists or counselors can equip you with coping mechanisms and emotional support.
- **Explore Community Resources:** Respite care services or in-home care options can provide temporary relief from caregiving duties.

Remember: Self-care is not selfish; it is an investment in your ability to care for yourself and others effectively. By prioritizing your well-being, managing stress, and seeking support, you can become a stronger, more resilient caregiver. You deserve to be taken care of too.

28. LEISURE, SOCIALIZATION, AND INCLUSION

Leisure activities and social interaction are essential ingredients in a fulfilling life for everyone, and individuals with disabilities are no exception. This chapter explores the importance of leisure and socialization, how to adapt activities for different needs, and strategies for facilitating community inclusion. Remember, everyone deserves opportunities to have fun, connect with others, and explore their interests.

Importance of Leisure Activities and Socialization

Engaging in leisure activities and socializing offers a multitude of benefits for individuals with disabilities:

- **Improved Mental Wellbeing:** Leisure activities can reduce stress, promote relaxation, and boost mood.
- **Enhanced Social Skills:** Social interaction helps develop communication skills, build friendships, and foster a sense of belonging.
- **Physical Activity:** Many leisure activities involve movement, contributing to physical health and well-being.
- **Increased Confidence:** Successfully participating in activities can build self-esteem and a sense of accomplishment.

- **Learning and Growth:** Leisure activities can provide opportunities for learning new skills and exploring interests.

Identifying and Adapting Leisure Activities for Different Needs and Abilities

The key to successful inclusion is adapting activities to individual needs. Here are some considerations:

- **Physical Limitations:** Modify activities to accommodate mobility limitations, sensory sensitivities, or other physical restrictions. For example, use adaptive equipment or choose seated activities.
- **Cognitive Abilities:** Select activities that fit the individual's cognitive level. Consider games with clear rules, structured activities, or opportunities for creative expression.
- **Interests:** Focus on activities the individual enjoys. This could be anything from sports and music to arts and crafts or spending time outdoors.

Facilitating Social Interactions and Community Integration

Promoting social interaction and community involvement is crucial. Here are some strategies:

- **Inclusive Environments:** Seek out inclusive programs and activities designed for individuals with diverse abilities.
- **Social Skills Training:** Programs can teach social communication skills, building confidence in social situations.
- **Peer Support Groups:** Connecting with others facing similar challenges can provide a sense of belonging and friendship opportunities.
- **Mentorship Programs:** Matching individuals with disabilities with mentors can provide guidance and social connection.

Transportation and Accessibility Considerations for Leisure Activities

Transportation and accessibility can be hurdles to participation. Here is how to overcome them:

- **Accessible Transportation:** Explore accessible public transport options or utilize paratransit services.
- **Planning and Preparation:** Research accessibility features of venues or activities beforehand to ensure a smooth experience.
- **Requesting Accommodations:** Do not be afraid to communicate accessibility needs to program organizers or event venues to ensure participation is possible.

Remember: Everyone deserves a chance to relax, have fun, and connect with others. By adapting activities, promoting inclusion, and addressing accessibility barriers, we can create a world where leisure and social interaction are possible for all. Let us encourage participation and celebrate the joy of shared experiences.

29. FINANCIAL PLANNING AND BENEFITS ASSISTANCE

Financial security is a cornerstone of a stable and fulfilling life. This chapter explores government benefits and assistance programs available for individuals with disabilities, along with essential financial planning considerations, estate planning tips, and valuable resources for further guidance. Remember, with knowledge and planning, you can build a secure financial future.

Government Benefits and Assistance Programs

Many government programs offer financial aid and support to individuals with disabilities. Here is a brief overview:

- **Social Security Disability Insurance (SSDI):** Provides monthly income for individuals with disabilities who are unable to work due to a medical condition.
- **Supplemental Security Income (SSI):** Provides financial assistance to individuals with disabilities who have limited income and resources.
- **Medicaid:** Provides health insurance coverage for low-income individuals and families, including those with disabilities.
- **Vocational Rehabilitation Services:** Provides resources to help individuals with disabilities

obtain job training, education, and employment opportunities.

It is important to note: Eligibility criteria and application processes can vary depending on your location and specific needs. Researching and seeking professional guidance can ensure you are receiving all the benefits you are entitled to.

Planning for the Future

Financial planning takes on a unique dimension for individuals with disabilities. Here are some key considerations:

- **Increased Expenses:** Disability-related costs, such as medical care, assistive technology, or transportation, can increase financial needs.
- **Employment Challenges:** Individuals with disabilities may face employment barriers, impacting income potential.
- **Long-Term Care Planning:** Consider the potential need for long-term care services and the associated costs.
- **Investment Strategies:** Invest for the future to manage expenses and secure financial stability. Seek professional financial advice for personalized investment strategies.

Estate Planning and Legal Considerations

Estate planning ensures your assets are distributed according to your wishes after your passing. It is particularly important for individuals with disabilities:

- **Special Needs Trusts:** These trusts can provide for the financial well-being of a beneficiary with a disability without jeopardizing their eligibility for government benefits.
- **Guardianship and Power of Attorney:** Consider appointing guardians to manage your finances and healthcare decisions if you are unable to do so in the future.

Resources for Financial Assistance and Advocacy

Numerous resources exist to assist with financial planning and advocacy for individuals with disabilities. Here are some examples:

- **Disability Rights Organizations:** These organizations provide information, advocacy, and legal assistance related to financial benefits and rights.
- **Government Agencies:** Many government agencies offer financial resources and planning tools specifically for individuals with disabilities.

- **Financial Advisors:** Seek a financial advisor specializing in planning for individuals with disabilities to create a personalized financial plan.

Remember: Financial planning is an ongoing process. By exploring government benefits, considering your unique needs, and seeking professional guidance, you can build a secure financial future and plan for a brighter tomorrow. You are not alone on this journey.

30. ADVOCACY AND EMPOWERMENT FOR INDIVIDUAL RIGHTS

Everyone deserves to have their voice heard and their rights upheld. This chapter delves into the importance of advocacy for individuals with disabilities. It explores the role of caregivers, self-advocacy skills development, effective communication with professionals, and navigating the legal landscape surrounding disability rights. Remember, empowerment starts with having a voice and knowing your rights.

Advocating for the Rights of People with Disabilities

Caregivers play a crucial role in advocating for the rights of individuals with disabilities. Here is how you can champion their cause:

- **Become an Informed Advocate:** Educate yourself about disability rights and relevant legislation. Familiarize yourself with the specific needs and goals of the individual you care for.
- **Empower Communication:** Support individuals in communicating their needs and preferences as much as possible.
- **Be a Liaison:** Collaborate with healthcare providers, educators, and other service providers to ensure the individual's rights and needs are met.

- **Speak Up When Needed:** If an individual's rights are disregarded, advocate on their behalf in a respectful and assertive manner.

Self-Advocacy Skills and Empowerment Training

Self-advocacy empowers individuals with disabilities to speak up for themselves and make informed decisions about their lives. Here is how to support self-advocacy development:

- **Communication Skills Training:** Programs can enhance communication skills, fostering clear expression of needs and desires.
- **Decision-Making Skills Development:** Activities can help individuals develop the confidence to make choices and manage their lives.
- **Disability Rights Education:** Learning about rights and resources empowers individuals to navigate the system more confidently.

Communication and Collaboration with Healthcare Providers and Educators

Effective communication with healthcare providers and educators is essential. Here are some tips:

- **Be Prepared:** Come to appointments with a list of concerns, questions, and desired outcomes.

- **Clear Communication:** Speak clearly and concisely about the individual's needs and preferences.
- **Collaborative Approach:** Work together with professionals to develop a care plan or educational program that fits the individual's needs.
- **Respectful Assertiveness:** Advocate for the individual's rights while maintaining respectful communication.

Navigating Legal Systems and Disability Rights Legislation

Understanding disability rights legislation empowers individuals to access services and opportunities. Here is how to navigate the legal landscape:

- **Research Relevant Laws:** Get familiar with laws like the Americans with Disabilities Act (ADA) or the Individuals with Disabilities Education Act (IDEA), which protect the rights of individuals with disabilities.
- **Seek Legal Guidance:** If you encounter discrimination or barriers, consider seeking legal advice or contacting disability rights organizations.
- **Advocacy Groups:** Many organizations offer resources and support to navigate legal challenges and advocate for equal access.

Remember: Empowerment starts with having a voice.

By advocating for the rights of individuals with disabilities, fostering self-advocacy skills, and navigating the legal landscape, we can create a world where everyone is empowered to reach their full potential.

31. BUILDING POSITIVE RELATIONSHIPS

The heart of caregiving lies in the relationship between the caregiver and the individual receiving care. This chapter explores the importance of building trust, respect, and understanding. We will discuss effective communication strategies, setting healthy boundaries, and fostering a supportive environment. Remember, a positive relationship is the foundation for quality care and a sense of well-being for both parties.

Building Trust and Respectful Relationships

A strong caregiver-care recipient relationship is built on trust and respect. Here is why it matters:

- **Improved Quality of Care:** Trust fosters open communication, leading to better understanding of needs and preferences.
- **Enhanced Well-being:** Respectful interactions create a positive environment, promoting emotional well-being for both caregiver and care recipient.
- **Increased Cooperation:** Trust fosters a sense of partnership, encouraging collaboration in care decisions.

Understanding the Individual's Preferences and Needs

Taking the time to understand the individual you care

for is crucial. Here is how to gain valuable insights:

- **Active Listening:** Pay close attention to their concerns, desires, and communication style.
- **Empathy:** Try to see things from their perspective and understand their emotional experiences.
- **Respecting Choices:** As much as possible, involve them in decisions about their care and daily routines.

Effective Communication Strategies for Building Rapport

Clear and respectful communication is vital. Here are some tips:

- **Simple and Direct Language:** Use clear, concise language that's easy to understand.
- **Active Listening:** Pay attention to both verbal and nonverbal cues.
- **Positive Reinforcement:** Acknowledge and praise cooperative behaviors and progress.
- **Open-Ended Questions:** Encourage conversation and expression of needs by asking open-ended questions.

Setting Healthy Boundaries and Maintaining Professionalism

Setting healthy boundaries protects both the caregiver and the care recipient from burnout and resentment. Here are some considerations:

- **Personal Time:** Schedule time for your own well-being to avoid caregiver fatigue.
- **Professional Limits:** Clearly define your role and responsibilities, avoiding tasks beyond your competence.
- **Maintaining Respect:** Treat the individual with respect and dignity, even in moments of frustration.

Providing Emotional Support and Encouragement

Emotional support is an essential aspect of caregiving. Here is how to offer encouragement:

- **Empathetic Listening:** Be a listening ear and validate their feelings.
- **Positive Reinforcement:** Acknowledge their strengths and celebrate their accomplishments.
- **Encouragement and Patience:** Support their independence and offer encouragement when facing challenges.

Remember: Building a positive relationship takes time and effort. By fostering trust, respect, understanding, and clear communication, you can create a supportive environment where both the caregiver and the care recipient can thrive.

32. EMERGENCY PREPAREDNESS AND FIRST AID

Emergencies can happen anytime, anywhere. This chapter emphasizes the importance of being prepared for individuals with disabilities. We will explore developing a personalized emergency plan, fire safety considerations, basic first aid training for caregivers, and disaster preparedness tips. Remember, a little planning can go a long way in ensuring everyone's safety in an emergency.

Planning for the Unexpected

A well-defined emergency plan provides peace of mind and ensures everyone knows what to do in an emergency. Here is what to consider:

- **Identify Evacuation Needs:** Plan escape routes that consider mobility limitations or sensory sensitivities. Include information on assistive devices needed during evacuation.
- **Communication Plan:** Determine how to communicate emergency information, such as using visual cues, alarms with vibrations, or text-to-speech devices.
- **Buddy System:** If necessary, assign a buddy to assist the individual with evacuation or communication during an emergency.

- **Emergency Contact Information:** Have a readily accessible list of emergency contacts, including healthcare providers and family members.
- **Practice Makes Perfect:** Regularly practice evacuation drills to familiarize everyone with the plan.

Fire Safety and Evacuation Procedures

Fire safety is paramount. Here are some fire safety tips for individuals with disabilities:

- **Install Smoke Alarms:** Ensure smoke alarms are functional and consider installing alarms with strobe lights for those with hearing impairments.
- **Clear Escape Routes:** Maintain clear escape routes free from clutter and ensure doorways are wide enough to accommodate assistive devices.
- **Evacuation Plan for Every Floor:** If living in a multi-story building, have an evacuation plan for each floor.

Basic First Aid and CPR Training for Caregivers

Basic first aid and CPR training can be lifesaving. Consider taking a course to be prepared for common emergencies:

- **Choking:** Learn the Heimlich maneuver for adults and children.
- **Wounds and Bleeding:** Know how to apply pressure and bandage wounds.
- **CPR:** Basic CPR skills can significantly improve survival rates in cardiac arrest situations.

Disaster Preparedness and Considerations for Different Disabilities

Disaster preparedness involves planning for various emergencies beyond fires. Here are some considerations for different disabilities:

- **Visual Impairments:** Provide tactile maps or braille instructions for evacuation routes.
- **Hearing Impairments:** Invest in visual fire alarms and ensure communication plans incorporate visual cues.
- **Mobility Limitations:** Identify accessible evacuation routes and consider having a battery-powered evacuation chair if needed.

Information Accessibility

Everyone deserves access to critical information during emergencies. Here is how to ensure accessibility:

- **Emergency Alert Systems:** Register for text message or visual alert systems that provide emergency information.
- **Accessible Websites:** Government websites and emergency management agencies should offer information in accessible formats like large print or audio recordings.
- **Sign Language Interpretation:** Ensure emergency briefings and public announcements include sign language interpretation.

Remember: Being prepared empowers individuals with disabilities and their caregivers to respond effectively in emergencies. By developing a plan, focusing on fire safety, acquiring basic first-aid skills, and ensuring information accessibility, we can create a safer environment for everyone.

33. END-OF-LIFE CARE CONSIDERATIONS

End-of-life care focuses on providing comfort and support to individuals and their loved ones facing a terminal illness. This chapter explores end-of-life care options for individuals with disabilities, pain management considerations, the importance of communication, and resources for grief and bereavement support. Remember, open communication and compassionate care can bring a sense of peace and dignity during this sensitive time.

Understanding End-of-Life Care Options for People with Disabilities

Individuals with disabilities deserve quality end-of-life care, tailored to their specific needs. Here is an overview of some options:

- **Hospice Care:** Provides comfort-focused care at home, in a hospice facility, or a hospital setting. It focuses on pain management, emotional support, and spiritual care.
- **Palliative Care:** Focuses on managing pain and symptoms of chronic illnesses, not just at the end of life. It can be provided alongside curative treatments.
- **Home Care:** Many people with disabilities may prefer to receive end-of-life care at home in familiar surroundings.

Providing Comfort and Support During End-of-Life Stages

Providing comfort and support goes beyond medical care. Here is how to show compassion:

- **Respecting Wishes:** Honor the individual's preferences regarding care options and level of intervention.
- **Emotional Support:** Be present, listen actively, and offer emotional support to the individual and family members.
- **Spiritual Care:** Respect and support the individual's spiritual or religious beliefs.

Pain Management and Palliative Care Considerations

Pain management is crucial for comfort at the end of life. Here is what to consider:

- **Communicating Pain Levels:** Individuals with disabilities may experience or express pain differently. Be attentive to subtle cues and encourage communication of discomfort.
- **Palliative Care Teams:** These teams specialize in managing pain and symptoms using medication, therapies, and other techniques.

- **Individualized Approach:** Pain management plans are tailored to the specific needs and medical conditions of the individual.

Communication with the Individual and Family Members about End-of-Life Wishes

Open and honest communication is essential during end-of-life planning. Here is how to facilitate communication:

- **Early Discussions:** Conversations about end-of-life wishes should happen well before a crisis.
- **Respecting Autonomy:** Support the individual's right to make decisions about their care.
- **Family Involvement:** Include family members in discussions and respect their perspectives.
- **Advance Directives:** Encourage the completion of advance directives, which document the individual's wishes for care in case they are unable to communicate them directly.

Grief and Bereavement Support for Caregivers and Family

The loss of a loved one is a deeply personal experience. Here is how to access support:

- **Grief Support Groups:** Connecting with others who have experienced similar loss can be a source of comfort and understanding.
- **Professional Counseling:** Consider seeking professional counseling to navigate the grieving process.
- **Self-Care:** Prioritize your own well-being during this difficult time. Engage in activities that bring you comfort and support.

Remember: End-of-life care is about respecting the individual's wishes and providing comfort during a difficult time. By understanding options, communicating openly, and offering compassionate care, we can create a sense of peace and dignity for everyone involved.

34. ETHICAL CONSIDERATIONS IN DISABILITY CARE

Disability care is a complex field, requiring a strong ethical foundation. This chapter explores essential principles like confidentiality, informed consent, and respecting diversity. We will discuss ethical dilemmas, the importance of cultural competency, and maintaining professional boundaries. Remember, ethical care ensures the dignity, autonomy, and well-being of the individual.

Maintaining Confidentiality and Privacy of the Individual

Confidentiality is paramount. Here is how to protect an individual's privacy:

- **Limited Disclosure:** Share information only with those directly involved in the individual's care.
- **Secure Records:** Maintain medical records and personal information in a secure and confidential manner.
- **Respecting Privacy:** Ask permission before discussing personal matters with others, even family members, unless required by law.

Obtaining Informed Consent for Care Decisions

Informed consent is crucial for respecting autonomy.

Here is what it entails:

- **Clear Communication:** Provide information about treatment options, potential risks and benefits, and alternative approaches in a clear and understandable way.
- **Assessing Understanding:** Ensure the individual understands the information before obtaining consent.
- **Respecting Choices:** Respect the right of the individual to make choices about their care, even if you disagree.

Ethical Dilemmas in Disability Care and Decision-Making Processes

Disability care can present ethical dilemmas. Here is how to navigate them:

- **Seeking Guidance:** Consult with colleagues, ethics committees, or healthcare professionals when facing complex decisions.
- **Balancing Interests:** Consider the best interests of the individual, respecting their autonomy while safeguarding their well-being.
- **Advocating for the Individual:** Be a strong advocate for the individual's rights and wishes, especially when dealing with complex situations or competing interests.

Cultural Competency and Respecting Diversity in Caregiving

Cultural competency involves understanding and respecting individual cultural backgrounds, beliefs, and values. Here is how to ensure culturally sensitive care:

- **Respecting Traditions:** Be mindful of cultural practices that may influence healthcare decisions or preferences.
- **Communication Styles:** Adapt communication methods to accommodate different cultural communication styles.
- **Avoiding Assumptions:** Do not make assumptions about beliefs or preferences based on cultural background.

Professional Boundaries and Avoiding Exploitation

Maintaining professional boundaries protects both the caregiver and the individual. Here is what to avoid:

- **Personal Relationships:** Avoid developing personal or romantic relationships with individuals receiving care.
- **Financial Exploitation:** Never use your position to gain financial advantage from the individual or their family.

- **Gifts and Favors:** Avoid accepting gifts or favors that could be perceived as compromising your professional judgment.

Remember: Ethical considerations are at the heart of quality care. By maintaining confidentiality, obtaining informed consent, respecting diversity, and upholding professional boundaries, we can ensure that individuals with disabilities receive care that is dignified, respectful, and empowers them to make their own choices.

35. GRIEF AND LOSS IN DISABILITY CARE

A disability diagnosis, for both the individual and the caregiver, can be a life-altering event. This chapter explores the grieving process, healthy coping mechanisms, and resources for navigating loss and change. Remember, grief is a natural response to loss, and support is available to help you through this journey.

Understanding the Grieving Process After a Disability Diagnosis

A disability diagnosis can trigger a grieving process similar to losing a loved one. Here is why:

- **Loss of Independence:** Individuals may grieve the loss of abilities or the life they envisioned for themselves.
- **Uncertain Future:** The unknown aspects of living with a disability can cause anxiety and fear.
- **Shifting Roles:** Caregivers may grieve the loss of their relationship with the individual before the diagnosis.

It is important to remember: The grieving process is unique for everyone. There is no right or wrong way to feel.

Coping Mechanisms for Dealing with Loss and Change

Healthy coping mechanisms can help navigate grief and adjust to change. Here are some strategies:

- **Allow Yourself to Grieve:** Do not suppress your emotions. Acknowledge your feelings and allow yourself to grieve.
- **Seek Support:** Talk to friends, family, therapists, or support groups about your experiences.
- **Focus on What You Can Control:** Focus on the aspects of life you can control and celebrate small victories.
- **Maintain a Healthy Lifestyle:** Prioritize sleep, exercise, and healthy eating habits to manage stress and improve well-being.

Supporting a Grieving Heart

- **Open Communication:** Create a safe space for open communication about their feelings and concerns.
- **Validation:** Validate their emotions and avoid minimizing their experiences.
- **Focus on Strengths:** Help them rediscover their strengths and abilities, fostering self-confidence.
- **Encourage Independence:** Support their independence as much as possible to maintain a sense of control.

Managing Caregiver Grief and Emotional Wellbeing

Caregivers also experience grief and emotional strain. Here is how to prioritize your well-being:

- **Acknowledge Your Feelings:** Do not feel guilty about grieving. Allow yourself to feel your emotions.
- **Seek Support:** Connect with other caregivers or therapists to share your experiences and find support.
- **Practice Self-Care:** Schedule time for activities you enjoy to avoid burnout. Prioritize sleep, relaxation, and healthy habits.
- **Set Boundaries:** Set healthy boundaries to protect your emotional well-being and avoid caregiver fatigue.

Support Groups and Resources for Coping with Loss

Numerous resources exist to help cope with loss and adjust to disability. Here are some examples:

- **Support Groups:** Connecting with others facing similar challenges can provide understanding and a sense of community.

- **Disability Organizations:** Many organizations offer resources and support programs for individuals with disabilities and their caregivers.
- **Mental Health Professionals:** Therapy can provide valuable tools and support for managing grief and emotional challenges.

Remember: Grief is a natural response to loss. By acknowledging your feelings, adopting healthy coping mechanisms, and seeking support, you can navigate this challenging journey. You are not alone. There are resources available to help you and the individual you care for move forward with strength and resilience.

36. GUARDIANSHIP, POWER OF ATTORNEY AND ADVANCE DIRECTIVES

Legal matters can be complex, especially when it comes to disability care. This chapter explores key legal concepts like guardianship, power of attorney, and advance directives. Understanding these tools can help ensure the well-being and decision-making rights of individuals with disabilities. Remember, legal guidance can empower you to make informed choices.

Guardianship and Conservatorship Laws for Individuals with Disabilities

Guardianship and conservatorship are legal processes that appoint someone to make decisions on behalf of an individual deemed unable to manage their own affairs. Here is a breakdown:

- **Guardianship:** Focuses on personal decisions like residence, healthcare, and daily living arrangements.
- **Conservatorship:** Focuses on financial decisions like managing assets and income.

It is important to note: Guardianship and conservatorship should only be considered when absolutely necessary. Least restrictive alternatives should be explored first.

Power of Attorney and Healthcare Proxies for Decision-Making

A power of attorney is a legal document that allows someone (the agent) to make decisions on another person's (the principal) behalf when they are unable to do so themselves. There are two main types:

- **Durable Power of Attorney:** Remains valid even if the principal becomes incapacitated.
- **Healthcare Proxy (or Medical Power of Attorney):** Specifically grants decision-making authority regarding medical treatment.

Advance Directives and Living Wills

An advance directive is a legal document that outlines an individual's wishes for future medical care in case they are incapacitated. It can include:

- **Living Will:** Specifies preferences regarding life-sustaining treatment.
- **Do Not Resuscitate (DNR) Order:** Instructs medical professionals to withhold CPR in case of cardiac arrest.

Advance directives are essential for ensuring your wishes are respected regarding end-of-life care.

Legal Advocacy and Access to Legal Services

Legal advocacy can be crucial for individuals with disabilities to protect their rights and access essential services. Here is what you should know:

- **Disability Rights Organizations:** Many organizations provide legal advocacy and resources for navigating legal processes related to disability.
- **Legal Aid:** Low-income individuals may qualify for legal aid services to assist with legal matters.
- **Estate Planning Attorneys:** Consider consulting an attorney specializing in estate planning for individuals with disabilities to create a comprehensive plan.

Remember: Legal matters can be complex, but understanding your options empowers you to make informed decisions. By exploring legal concepts like guardianship, power of attorney, and advance directives, and seeking guidance if needed, you can ensure that the individual's rights and wishes are protected.

37. PLANNING FOR LONG-TERM NEEDS AND RESIDENTIAL OPTIONS

As we age, our needs may change. This chapter explores planning for long-term care for individuals with disabilities. We will delve into residential options, transitioning to new living arrangements, technological advancements, financial considerations, and resources to ensure a secure and fulfilling future. Remember, proactive planning empowers you to make informed choices about your care as you age.

Looking Ahead

Early planning for long-term care needs is crucial. Here is what to consider:

- **Individual Needs:** Assess the current and potential future needs of the individual, considering physical limitations and independence level.
- **Support Systems:** Evaluate available support systems from family, friends, or paid caregivers.
- **Financial Resources:** Explore potential funding options for long-term care, including government benefits, personal savings, and insurance.
- **Desired Lifestyle:** Consider the individual's preferences for living arrangements and desired level of independence.

Types of Residential Options

There is a spectrum of residential options available, each offering varying levels of support. Here is an overview:

- **Independent Living:** Individuals live in their own homes or apartments with minimal or no assistance with daily activities.
    - o Often includes accessible housing modifications and in-home care services.
- **Assisted Living:** Offers private apartments with assistance with daily living activities like meals, bathing, and medication management.
    - o Provides a supportive environment with social and recreational activities.
- **Nursing Homes:** Provide 24/7 skilled medical care for individuals who require a high level of assistance.

It is important to note: The best option depends on the individual's specific needs and preferences. Flexibility and adaptability are key as needs may change over time.

Transition Planning and Considerations for Aging with a Disability

Transitioning to a new living arrangement can be stressful. Here is how to ensure a smooth move:

- **Involve the Individual:** Include the individual in discussions and planning for their future living situation.
- **Gradual Adjustments:** Consider trial stays or short-term visits to help with adaptation.
- **Familiarization Visits:** Organize visits to potential residential facilities to ease anxiety and promote familiarity.
- **Maintaining Connections:** Help the individual stay connected with loved ones to combat feelings of isolation.

Technological Advancements and Assistive Technologies for Future Care

Technology is revolutionizing care for individuals with disabilities. Here are some potential benefits:

- **Smart Homes:** Technology can automate tasks like lighting, temperature control, and door locks, promoting independence.
- **Assistive Devices:** Wearable health monitors, robotic assistants, and voice-activated controls can enhance safety and independence.
- **Telehealth:** Remote access to healthcare providers through video conferencing can improve access to care.

Financial Planning and Funding Options

Long-term care can be expensive. Here is how to prepare financially:

- **Government Benefits:** Explore programs like Medicaid and veterans' benefits that may offer assistance with long-term care costs.
- **Long-Term Care Insurance:** Consider purchasing long-term care insurance to help offset future costs.
- **Financial Planning Professionals:** Seek guidance from a financial advisor specializing in long-term care planning.

Remember: Planning for long-term care empowers individuals with disabilities to maintain their independence and well-being as they age. By exploring residential options, considering future needs, and embracing technological advancements, you can build a secure and fulfilling future.

Can You Help Others Find This Book by Writing a Review?

Thank you for reading the book. As a retired physician with a fresh viewpoint, I am dedicating my time to creating this informative series out of a desire to empower others through credible information. This series is my way of continuing to serve others, not for profit, but out of a deep love and passion for sharing knowledge to benefit those who are perplexed by the overwhelming information overload in the digital world. Therefore, I have created this series of patient information books as a one-stop information haven, painstakingly built to save you valuable time. Your honest review on Amazon, accessible through the QR code below, will be a guiding light for others seeking clarity. Let us empower each other, one informed reader at a time! Kindly write a review about this book!

ABOUT THE AUTHOR

Dr. A. Mitra is a retired medical doctor who has worked in the field of General Practice in Family Medicine in India and Australia for over 30 years. He completed his graduate education in India and then did further studies in Australia and UK. Currently he lives a private modest life and pursues his interests in reading and writing on various topics.